Coping
With an
Ostomy

A GUIDE TO LIVING WITH AN OSTOMY
FOR YOU AND YOUR FAMILY

Coping
With an
Ostomy

ROBERT H. PHILLIPS, Ph.D.

AVERY PUBLISHING GROUP INC.
Wayne, New Jersey

Cover design by Martin Hochberg
In-house editor Jacqueline Balla
Designed by Diana Puglisi
Typesetting by ACS Graphic Services, Fresh Meadows, NY

Library of Congress Cataloging-in-Publication Data

Phillips, Robert H., 1948–
  Coping with an ostomy.

  Bibliography: p.
  Includes index.
  1. Ostomates--Psychology. 2. Ostomates--Care and
treatment. 3. Enterostomy--Social aspects. I. Title.
RD540.P47   1986   617'.55   85-22810
ISBN 0-89529-277-7 (pbk.)

Printed in the United States of America

10 9 8 7 6 5 4 3 2 1

Contents

Dedication

This book is lovingly dedicated to my family: my wife, Sharon, and my three sons, Michael, Larry, and Steven; my parents, sister, and grandparents, as well as my other relatives and in-laws.

In addition, this book is gratefully dedicated to those wonderful people, friends as well as family, who have been there for me, both to provide love and support when I needed it, and to enjoy sharing progress and growth. Thanks.

Acknowledgements

Grateful words of thanks must be communicated to some wonderful people, who provided invaluable assistance in the preparation of this book. Thanks to Naomi Laughton, R.N., E.T., whose friendship and expertise have been such assets, not only to me, but to thousands of others, and whose critical review was so helpful. Thanks to Ellen Maye for the hours spent efficiently transcribing, revising, and editing the manuscript. Thanks to Pamela DiStefano and Shelley Markowitz for their help in transcription. Thanks to Lawrence Greene, M.D., and Sidney Fierst, M.D., for introducing me to the world of the ostomate, and to Ralph Feller, Harold Rosenblaum, and Rob Schildkraut, for making me feel like such an important part of the Ostomy Association of Brooklyn and the Long Island Ostomy Association. Thanks to my publisher, Rudy Shur, who has been so encouraging (both in the writing of the book and in reminding me not to forget him in the acknowledgements!). Finally, thanks to Joyce Stein, R.N., E.T., for her personal and professional guidance, encouragement, and support, and for being such an inspiration to me, as well as to so many countless professionals, colleagues, ostomates, and others.

Foreword

Why me? What did I do to deserve this? How could it happen? That's the end of my life. I'd rather be dead! How often have these questions been asked, and those desperate statements made!

When we realize that, in the United States alone, there are over 100,000 people each year who will be undergoing surgery to create an ostomy, how can we not think about the anguish and anxiety that this procedure will provoke? Certainly, it's comforting that self-help groups have come into existence to answer the need for a supportive, sharing-caring experience, and that ostomy chapters throughout the world have played leading roles in the rehabilitation of the person with an ostomy.

This need was acknowledged again when, much more recently, a new nursing specialty was created, called the enterostomal therapist. This is a nurse who has attended an accredited training program preparing her to provide care and expertise to the person undergoing ostomy surgery. As a member of this profession personally, I cannot speak highly enough of their contributions and dedication towards every aspect of the ostomate. Their roles are multi-faceted, for there are many sub-titles that are pertinent and specific towards the basic goal of total rehabilitation of the patient with a stoma.

When we have been damaged, accepting a less than perfect "me" is not easy. As we start the process of rebuilding, we need to call upon our coping mechanisms to help us regain and renew the way we view ourselves. Today we are fortunate because there are numerous support systems available, helping to make the transition smoother and, hopefully, faster. It is my opinion that one should call upon and utilize as many of these systems as necessary to achieve this goal. They must do whatever is need-ed to again create a sense of worth to themselves, their family and friends, and to once again become active participants in society. To live a life of dignity and to feel socially acceptable is entirely possible with an ostomy, if it is your desire to make it so. The choice is yours.

A very important tool in the supportive process is the written word. Verbal input, teaching, visual aids, and ostomy volunteer visits are quite necessary and vital to a new ostomate. However, material to read, absorb, or refer to is also essential. Patients are constantly asking me for literature to use for reference, reassurance, and information. When Dr. Phillips told me he was contemplating writing a book for ostomates, I was thrilled. In the years that I've known Bob Phillips, he has been an active contributor to ostomy clubs and seminars as a speaker and panelist participant. He has shown a most sincere interest in the concerns and problems of the ostomate. As a practicing psychologist, he is very well qualified to offer compassionate advice and information that will undoubtedly quicken the process towards a better quality of life.

I have lived with an ostomy for well over two decades and, therefore, speak from "both sides of the bed"; as an ostomate and as an enterostomal therapist. I have never said that having an ostomy is wonderful. I do know that, with good preparation and teaching, life with one can be very livable and has truly given me a marvelous gift of life. Dr. Phillips has pro-vided us with a comprehensive resource filled with excellent information, to make living with a stoma much more acceptable than we may have thought possible. I am grateful to him for having the insight, the interest, and the desire to skillfully design a route to reach that acceptance.

Joyce Stein, R.N., E.T.
Enterostomal Therapist
Nurse Practitioner
Long Island Jewish-Hillside Medical Center
New Hyde Park, NY

Preface

An ostomy can have a major impact on you and your family. No kidding! Ostomies can cause an emotional reaction rarely seen with other chronic problems. Why? Your body has changed, your "plumbing" has changed, and you'll have all kinds of thoughts related to removal of part of your waste elimination system. Upon being diagnosed, many questions may come to mind. Physicians and professionals may be able to answer some of them. Others may not be answerable, and this can be upsetting. Also, it can be upsetting to realize that this is happening to you. You may be reluctant to talk about it because you feel it sets you apart from others. Knowing that you have an ostomy can be depressing.

Surgical procedures used in creating ostomies have improved year by year. At the present time, these operations are relatively safe procedures. Therefore, from a medical point of view, the procedure may help you to feel better and to improve the quality of your life significantly. But what about the psychological effects of having an ostomy? Will it interfere with your previous lifestyle? A major factor, therefore, in determining how normal and emotionally stable your life will be is how well you cope with the unique aspects of having an ostomy.

Powerful stuff? It certainly is, but now you know why this book has been written. It is loaded with facts, suggestions, techniques, strategies, and other useful ideas. It was written specifically to help you (whether you've already had your surgery or are preparing for it), members of your family, and friends. The first part of the book presents background information on ostomies: what they are, what kinds of ostomies there are, some of the causes of ostomy surgery, what may occur during and after the surgery itself, details about equipment, and so on. The other main parts deal with different aspects of living with an ostomy, including coping with emotions, changes in lifestyle, and living with others. These are all important aspects of coping with an ostomy. We will explore them in detail, and you'll read suggestions and strategies, as well as illustrative case examples, for each component.

Remember: each person is unique. Even though a lot of similarities exist, your ostomy, as well as the way you experience it, will not be exactly like anyone else's. Therefore, it will be up to you to use the suggestions and strategies in this book to help you to cope as well as you possibly can. You may be unique, but by reading about how other ostomates adjust you'll see that you're not alone. Others do share a lot of what you feel. This can be very reassuring. Finally, remember that an ostomy is a procedure that changes part of your body, hopefully to rectify an illness, disease, or condition. It is a totally manageable phenomenon!

Until that time when modern medicine is able to create techniques and medications to eliminate the need for ostomy surgery, ostomies will continue to exist. Now you have one. It has been said that it takes an average of one year to adjust to ostomy surgery, including post-operative healing, training, and lifestyle adjustment. It is hoped that this book will help you to cope with it during this year and long thereafter, as well as help members of your family to cope.

Robert H. Phillips, Ph.D.
Center for Coping With Chronic Conditions
Garden City, NY

PART I

Ostomy—Some Background

1

What is an Ostomy?

Jack, a 46-year-old father of four, went to his doctor for a check-up. He had been feeling a little run-down recently, and had become concerned when he noticed blood in his stool. After a complete physical and extensive tests, his physician was now preparing to discuss the results in his consultation room. Jack, appearing somewhat ashen-faced and shaken, sat in the chair next to the desk. The doctor looked at him, and wasted no time in telling him, "Jack, you're going to need a colostomy." Panicky, Jack responded, "I'm going to need a *what?*"

Carole was a 26-year-old marketing researcher. She had been suffering through months of pain and diarrhea because of Crohn's disease, a chronic illness marked by inflammation along the digestive tract. She had seen a number of different physicians and tried several different treatments in an attempt to alleviate her agony. Finally, she went to a gastroenterologist who specialized in Crohn's. After a complete physical and extensive tests, the physician met with her in his consultation room, and wasted no time in telling her, "Carole, you're going to need an ileostomy." Trembling, Carole shrieked, "I'm going to need a *what?*"

Harry had been troubled by increasing difficulty in urinating. He started noticing pain in the area as well. He consulted a urologist, who completed a thorough examination and wasted no time in telling him, "Harry, you're going to need a urostomy." Harry collapsed into a chair and weakly voiced, "I'm going to need a *what?*"

Colostomy, ileostomy, urostomy. More and more people are recognizing these words, even if they don't yet recognize the word ostomy. But colostomy, ileostomies, and urostomies are three specific *types* of ostomies, and are, therefore, the focus of this book. So enough of an introduction already! What is an ostomy?

An ostomy is an artificial opening made surgically in the body. Ostomies can be placed in virtually any part of the body. This book, however, will focus on ostomies in the abdomen. Elimination of body wastes now takes place through this opening in the abdominal wall. The waste flows into a special appliance that is attached to this opening.

The word ostomy was originally used as a suffix. The first part of the word indicated the location of the ostomy. In other words, the colostomy is a surgical procedure involving the colon, the ileostomy involving the small intestine (or ileum), and the urostomy involving the urinary tract. Today, however, the word ostomy is used as a general term including these three types of procedures.

An ostomy is part of you. It is part of your body. It is not an illness. It is not a disease. It is not a condition. It is part of your "state of being," much the same as your navel, your elbow, or your fingernails are part of you. It may have resulted from an illness, a disease, or a condition, but it is now a physical part of you. Technically, this means that you are now an "ostomate." An ostomate is the person with the ostomy. (In England, the person is usually called an "ostomist." I wonder, any relation to optimist?)

Do you object to being called an ostomate? If you do, you're not alone. But remember that, first, you are a person, and second, you happen to have an ostomy. This emphasizes you, the person, rather than just identifying you as an ostomate. In actuality, most people with ostomies only call themselves ostomates when they are with others who have ostomies (such as at meetings).

WHY AN OSTOMY?

Body waste (urine and feces) must be eliminated from the body in order for it to continue to function properly. (A build-up of natural resources is desirable; a build-up of natural wastes is not!) So what happens if something interferes with this natural elimination process? Eureka, an ostomy may be the result! The ostomy provides an alternate way of eliminating body waste, either in the intestinal or urinary tract, if another condition or situation makes this necessary. In other words, an ostomy as a surgical procedure is usually performed when an individual has lost the ability to eliminate body waste through normal channels. Methods that you previously used to eliminate body waste may no longer be practical or possible. Maybe an accident or an injury occurred, damaging the intestine. Maybe an illness required a change in your plumbing, or a birth defect affected the elimination process. We will discuss this in more detail in the chapter, *Causes of Ostomy Surgery*.

LET'S STEP BACK A LITTLE

More and more people are hearing about ostomies today, but it was not always this way. As recently as twenty years ago, very few people knew what ostomies were. They weren't exactly popular subjects for conversation (really, now!) and few ostomates even admitted aloud that they had one. Now the ostomy seems to be coming out of the closet (the appliance closet?).

In the past, even nurses and other professionals involved in caring for the patient were not as familiar with ostomies or their care requirements. It's only recently that the specialty of enterostomal therapy (E.T.'s) has been established. E.T.'s are individuals with specialized training to handle the needs, both physical and psychological, of the ostomate.

WHO HAS OSTOMIES?

Ostomies are not rare. As a matter of fact, one and a half million Americans are estimated as having ostomies of different types. In addition, more than 100,000 ostomy operations are performed each year in the United States and Canada alone. Some of these ostomies are temporary, meaning that the diversion of waste to the abdominal opening may not necessarily be permanent. The original passageways may be reconnected so that elimination can proceed as before.

How old are ostomates? No one particular age seems to be the "winner" because ostomy surgery can be performed as early as minutes after birth up to the latest stages in life (the "seniors"). However, one noticeable finding is that, in general, it seems that more women have ostomy surgery than men.

TYPES OF OSTOMY SURGERY

As you learned from Jack, Carole, and Harry, we will be discussing three main categories of ostomy surgery: colostomies, ileostomies, and urostomies. Colostomies are performed when there's a problem with the colon (large intestine). The working part of the colon is brought to the new, surgically made opening, usually in a lower part of the abdomen. In ileostomies, the entire large intestine is bypassed (and usually removed). Then the end of the small intestine (the ileum) is also brought to the abdominal wall. However, the new opening is usually higher up than the opening for a colostomy might be. Urostomies involve surgical openings allowing urine to be eliminated from the body. Here, the ureter may be brought to the abdominal opening or, as in the case of a procedure called an ileal conduit, a piece of small intestine may be used to carry urine to the opening.

Colostomies are more common than either ileostomies or urostomies in adults. It is estimated that approximately two-thirds of all abdominal ostomies are colostomies. The older the adult, the more likely that the ostomy surgery will be a colostomy. This is usually because of cancer or obstruction-related problems. Ileostomies are more common in young adults, resulting from Crohn's disease or related intestinal disorders. Urostomies are more common in infants and the elderly. Of the non-colostomy ostomies, twice as many ileostomies are performed than urostomies.

OPENING UP TO THE STOMA

We've been talking a lot about the abdominal opening. It has a name. The stoma is the mouth or opening of the ostomy. Some ostomates give the stoma their own nickname. Such names as "Rosebud," "Oscar," "Herbie," or other terms of endearment are not uncommon. This may even help you to cope better. But please, don't talk to your stoma in a public place. And if you receive an answer . . . !

The surgeon usually brings a piece of the intestine through the abdominal wall, rolls it over, and sews it back on the abdominal wall. This stoma is mucousy and red in color because it is actually part of the intestine. It is flexible and soft. It acts as a type of valve, because it stretches to allow waste materials to pass through and out of the body. When not in use, it may shrink or pucker as it pulls together. This is similar to the way the anus pulls together when it's not being used. It may look similar to lips that are puckered for kissing! (Don't get any ideas!)

Although the stoma does stretch, expand, and contract, it does not contain the muscles that would do what the anal sphincter muscles do. So, unfortunately, it doesn't have the same ability to control or stop waste matter from flowing out of the body. It is, therefore, necessary to have some type of receptacle to catch this uncontrollable flow of waste. These receptacles, called appliances or pouches, are used to catch waste when it leaves the stoma. Other methods of waste control are also used. Some ostomates use irrigation as a way of regularly flushing out the large intestine. This is usually possible only with colostomies where the feces are more formed. There is another situation in which appliances are not necessary. Continent ileostomies involve the formation of a reservoir within the abdomen. This reservoir stores the waste and is then emptied by inserting a plastic tube through the stoma. More about all of this in the chapter, *Types of Ostomy Surgery*.

The stoma remains puffy following surgery, but this puffiness decreases slightly as time goes by. The diameter of the stoma (the width of the actual opening) may also decrease slightly. Despite changes in size, however, the red color remains. This is not a sign of inflammation; rather, it is the natural color of the intestinal wall's interior.

The size and shape of your stoma are unique. The stoma can also vary in both diameter and shape at different times. Stoma size and shape also depend on the type of ostomy surgery you have had, and on your own unique physical characteristics. Stomas range in size from smaller than a dime, to much larger than a half dollar. Some stomas are round, some are oval, some may be irregularly shaped. How far the stoma itself protrudes from the abdominal wall also depends on the type of ostomy performed. Colostomies usually have stomas that protrude only slightly from the abdominal wall, as little as a quarter of an inch. In ileostomies or urostomies the stoma sticks out further from the skin, since the consistency of waste is less formed (and, of course, urine is not formed at all). The stoma, looking something like a nipple, may protrude as much as three-fourths of an inch to an inch. Why? So the waste can easily flow into the attached receptacle, with less chance of irritation or damage from leakage to the skin surrounding the stoma.

The shape and size of the stoma should remain fairly constant once post-surgical swelling has gone down. However, if you either gain or lose a lot of weight, or become pregnant, this may alter the shape or contour of the stoma. If you notice a change in its color or shape without one of the above-mentioned causes, it might be a good idea to consult your physician.

Is The Stoma Fragile?

Soft and red. These are two adjectives describing the appearance of the stoma, which make it seem delicate. But the stoma is pretty hardy. It may bleed easily because blood vessels are always close to the walls of the intestines. If the stoma does bleed (even a gentle touch may cause this), it usually stops quickly. If the bleeding does not stop right away, applying ice should help. If this does not work, however, check with your physician.

With proper protection, the stoma can handle practically all of the abuses that normal skin does, other than bleeding. Although protection is necessary, you need not be obsessed with this. Stomas are not harmed by water, nor is sexual activity restricted. Gentle bumps will not create any damage, but jarring contact should be avoided, if possible. One of the surprising things about your stoma is that you will not feel pain. That's because the intestinal walls do not contain nerve endings. Even if you scratch or damage your stoma (accidentally, I assume!), you will not feel it. You may feel a sensation from the skin surrounding the stoma because there are nerve endings present. Yet, not being able to feel any damage is another reason why you should be careful to protect the stoma.

A stoma does not need to be washed, although many people feel comfortable giving it a gentle sponge bath. Showering or bathing is okay for the most part. Appliances or coverings are usually not necessary. Because of the movement of the intestines and the valve-like functioning of the stoma, water will not get back inside just because you're taking a shower or bath.

Stoma Surprises

Your stoma will discharge mucous. Knowing this will prevent surprise if you see this happening. Your intestines are mucousy by nature; mucous is simply the thick liquid that protects the lining of the intestinal wall. It also lubricates and enables the smooth passage of waste material. It's understandable, therefore, that excess mucous may seep out of your stoma.

Normally, waste moves smoothly through the intestine. Thank you, peristalsis. Peristalsis is the rhythmic contracting and expanding of the intestine. It keeps waste moving in the right direction. This peristaltic movement may bring you another surprise. There may be times when your stoma appears to be moving! But don't worry—your stoma is not trying to talk to you.

WHAT ABOUT THE FUTURE?

To get an idea of what the future will hold involves knowing what caused your ostomy surgery in the first place. But as far as ostomy surgery itself is concerned, prognosis has been improving significantly over the last fifteen to twenty years. Ostomy operations have become so routinely successful that survival rates have increased from less than 80% (fifteen to twenty years ago) to better than 97% (now). What accounts for this? Increasing expertise of physicians, improvements in equipment, and intensive research concerning gastrointestinal and urinary problems can all be thanked.

2

Causes of Ostomy Surgery

Why did you need ostomy surgery? *Why?* There are many possible reasons for such surgery. How do doctors decide? Let's talk about some of the diagnostic procedures used.

DIAGNOSING THE NEED

Different diagnostic tests are useful in helping physicians determine if surgery is necessary. These tests are performed either at the time of a regular medical examination in a doctor's office, or in a diagnostic center, lab, or hospital.

Radiology

The first category of diagnostic tests is that of the radiology tests. These usually involve the ingestion (taken orally or rectally) or injection (you'll get the point) of some type of liquid or dye. Whether this fluid is ingested or injected depends on what body system is being evaluated. If the problem concerns your intestines, then you'll probably ingest the liquid. If there is a urinary problem, then the liquid or dye may be injected.

One type of liquid used is barium. Chalk-flavored barium (delicious!) is ingested in one of two ways, depending on where in the intestines the problem is. The barium is swallowed by mouth if the upper gastrointestinal tract is being examined. Otherwise, it is introduced (glad to meet you) rectally, using an enema tube, if the lower gastrointestinal tract is being explored. Once the barium is inside the body, x-rays are taken. Hopefully, the diagnostician will be able to come up with an answer. What may be seen in these X-rays? They may diagnose lesions (damage to tissue or body part), polyps (little growths that don't belong), fistulae (openings or ulcers), or diverticuli (pouches or pockets in the intestinal wall). All are problems that could lead to ostomy surgery.

Once surgery has been performed, you'll probably return to the hospital or an out-patient clinic fairly frequently to repeat the examinations. This is to make sure that no complications have arisen. Your current condition may also be evaluated through ongoing barium tests. Once the ostomy is functioning, guess where the barium will go into your body? That's right, through your stoma, rather than through the rectum (especially if your rectum has been removed). "Isn't that much better?" you may ask. Not necessarily. In rectal enemas your anal muscles can retain the fluid better, so there will be more time for taking X-rays. But if your rectum has been removed, it will be very difficult for your stoma to retain fluid without these muscles. It may leak onto the abdominal wall surrounding it. What does this mean? Much more caution (not to mention faster-moving physicians!) is necessary.

What else may be injected into the body for diagnosis? If you're having problems with your urinary tract, an IVU (intravenous urogram) may be an appropriate diagnostic test. A dye is injected so that X-rays can determine whether there are problems with the bladder, kidneys, ureters, or any other urinary equipment.

Coping with Scopes

Another way of diagnosing the need for ostomy surgery is by "looking inside" your intestinal tract. This doesn't mean that your doctor has incredibly long, narrow eyeballs! Rather, this is done using *endoscopy*. Endoscopy procedures involve inserting tools or equipment through openings in the body (either natural openings or artificially created openings, such as stomas). The tools are used to visually diagnose problems that may exist. Occasionally, a camera may be attached to the endoscope, allowing photographs to be taken while the tube is inside the body (smile!). Sometimes, treatment can take place at the same time.

What is being investigated? The procedure enables the physician to detect any bleeding, growths, or changes in the bowel. Different types of endoscopy equipment are used for different parts of the intestine. You've probably heard some of the names. For example, the sigmoidoscope is used to explore the sigmoid part of the colon. Although not the most pleasant of diagnostic procedures, they are invaluable for what they're able to discover. Let's move on to some different reasons for ostomy surgery.

CANCER

Cancer is one of the most frequent causes of ostomy surgery. The location of the cancer determines which type of ostomy is necessary. The surgery is done either to stop the growth of cancerous cells, or because of the danger of tumor-causing obstructions or blockages. Tumors in the rectum, large, or small intestine may necessitate removal of all or part of the affected intestine. Cancer is also one of the more common reasons for a permanent urinary diversion, or urostomy. Tumors may result in the removal of the affected urinary part, such as the bladder or even the genitals.

Cancer does not always necessitate ostomy surgery. Efforts may be made first to fight the cancer non-surgically, using radiation, chemotherapy, or other methods. However, in cases where these procedures are unable to control the development of cancer or the recurrence of tumors, ostomy surgery may be necessary.

INFLAMMATORY BOWEL DISEASE

Inflammatory bowel disease (IBD) is not really one disease. Rather, it includes a number of illnesses or conditions in the intestinal tract. There are two main inflammatory bowel diseases that may lead to ostomy surgery: chronic ulcerative colitis and Crohn's disease. These are usually painful, prolonged intestinal conditions which, if other treatments are ineffective, may be completely and thankfully eliminated by ostomy surgery.

Ulcerative Colitis

Inflammatory bowel disease that affects the colon is called colitis. The most common form of colitis, in chronic form, is ulcerative colitis. This condition usually begins in the rectum and spreads upward through the large intestine, breaking up the inner walls of the large intestine in the process. The mucous lining of the large intestine may be destroyed. This can cause bloody diarrhea, and the ulcers in the intestine may necessitate ostomy surgery.

Ulcerative colitis is usually experienced in a roller-coaster way. If you've had it, you've probably gone through a series of remissions and exacerbations (or ups and downs). You probably had some of the more common symptoms, such as diarrhea, abdominal pain, bleeding, weight loss, and vomiting. Bowel movements are usually accompanied by blood and fluid loss. Doctors still don't know the condition's cause, and no cures exist yet. Ulcerative colitis usually attacks the large intestine, although occasionally the end of the small intestine may be involved. Medication is the primary type of treatment. When this fails, however, ostomy surgery may be necessary, requiring the removal of at least part of the colon. If that doesn't stop the illness, the entire large intestine may be removed, along with the rectum. The result? An ileostomy. It's important to treat chronic ulcerative colitis aggressively. Why? There is a higher risk of cancer in those who have the disease for long periods of time (usually ten years or more).

Crohn's Disease

Crohn's disease is an extremely painful, complex inflammatory bowel disease, most commonly affecting teenagers and young adults. It has several different names. When it affects the lower portion of the small intestine, it's also called ileitis. When it involves more of the intestine or a few different parts, it may be called regional enteritis. Other names for Crohn's disease, such as transmural entercolitis, are also used occasionally. (This doesn't include the names you'd like to call it if you've suffered from it!) How much of the intestine will be affected? There is no way of knowing whether the entire intestine will be involved or just parts of it. Actually, Crohn's disease may be found anywhere along the digestive tract (alimentary canal). So when would surgery be necessary? Crohn's may lead to ostomy surgery if the intestine is badly damaged, if scar tissue results in intestinal blockage, or if no other way has been effective in alleviating its painful symptoms.

INJURY OR ACCIDENT

Certain serious injuries or accidents may necessitate immediate ostomy surgery. A stabbing, for example, where the intestine is penetrated, or a gunshot, where the bullet perforates the intestine, may lead to ostomy surgery. An auto accident may also be the cause, if intestinal or urinary tract damage requires an alternate way of eliminating waste. Fortunately, many of these ostomies may be temporary. You may only need them until the injury is healed. Once healing is complete, additional surgery may be able to reconnect natural pathways for the elimination of waste.

If injury to the abdominal area or pelvis is very severe, the normal restoration of its function may be impossible. In this case, the ostomy will be permanent. What if an accident or a spinal injury damages or severs nerves? You might be paralyzed in the lower part of your body. Your bladder or bowel might be affected, and an ostomy may be necessary.

FAMILIAL POLYPOSIS

This condition is a hereditary one, in which many polyps grow in the intestine. There is a very high risk of cancer in such cases. Youngsters who develop familial polyposis may need to have their entire intestines removed to prevent the development of this cancer. Because familial polyposis is hereditary, it is essential that all members of the immediate family be carefully checked and monitored. Surgery in other family members may also be necessary.

SPINA BIFIDA

Spina bifida is a congenital birth defect which may, in some cases, create a need for ostomy surgery. In this condition, an opening in the infant's spine leaves the spinal cord unprotected. It is estimated that approximately six thousand babies per year are born with spina bifida. The condition has no known cause. Unfortunately, an infant born with spina bifida frequently has problems with either the bowel, the bladder, or both. Bowel problems may lead to colostomies. Peristalsis, necessary to move the feces through the intestine, may be weak or ineffective. Constipation, blockage, or impaction may result.

Ostomies may also result from bladder problems. In some cases, the bladder will not empty because of the condition. Retained fluid causes it to swell, and becomes much more susceptible to infection. On the other hand, the bladder may not be able to hold urine. It may spasm and frequently eliminate urine. Urostomy surgery may be necessary for more control. Up until recently, the vast majority of individuals born with spina bifida had ostomies (especially urostomies). Advances in medicine, resulting in better treatment, have reduced this number.

OTHER BIRTH DEFECTS

There are other birth defects that may necessitate ostomy surgery. Sometimes this surgery will be performed during infancy. In other cases, the birth defect may not become apparent until the child is older. Obviously, if surgery is necessary, it will also occur later.

Which birth defects can give rise to ostomy surgery? One is called neonatal necrotizing enterocolitis. In this condition, part of the bowel does not function. There may be dead tissue that doesn't allow waste material to pass through. This occurs most often in premature infants or in newborns weighing less than three pounds. However, this is not a common problem. Diagnosis can usually be made early and an ileostomy, often a temporary one, is a life-saver. When the infant grows older, it's likely that the intestines can be reconnected to function naturally. The ileostomy can then be eliminated.

Another birth defect that may result in ostomy surgery is an imperforate anus. The infant with this condition has an anus with no opening. There is no way for waste material to exit the body once it reaches the lower end of the intestine. If the problem is diagnosed early, a colostomy may be a temporary procedure, lasting until the imperforate anus condition can be corrected surgically. In some cases, however, bowel control may never be re-achieved and the colostomy may have to be permanent.

Are these the only birth defects leading to ostomy surgery? No. Others include conditions where nerves in the descending colon may be missing. Peristaltic activity would then break down. As a result, waste would not pass through this section of the intestine. Birth defects where the bladder forms outside of the body (called exstrophy of the bladder) usually necessitates urostomy surgery. There are also urinary conditions where excess tissue in the urinary tract prevents elimination. These may require ostomies as either temporary or permanent alternatives. Years of leakage or dripping in the urinary tract may also lead to urostomy surgery to resolve the problem.

A FINAL CAUSE PAUSE

There are many different reasons for ostomy surgery. These are the more common ones. However, there are cases where ostomies will result from diverticulitis (a condition known for its tearing or destruction of walls of the intestines), neurological disorders (where the bladder or bowel may be uncontrollable or may work in inappropriate fashion), formation of fistulae (abnormal openings within organs or parts of the body), or excessive growth of tissue.

The cause of the surgery obviously determines the kind of ostomy you'll end up with. The next chapter deals with the types of ostomy surgery in much more detail.

3

Types of Ostomy Surgery

In Chapter 1, Jack needed a colostomy. Carole needed an ileostomy. Harry needed a urostomy. These are the three main types of ostomy surgery. They all involve the creation of an artificial abdominal opening, through which waste matter can be eliminated from the body. By now you know why this is necessary, right? When natural elimination, either urination or defecation, cannot take place due to injury or illness, another route is necessary.

Depending upon the disease or the complexity of the condition, surgery may result in either a temporary or permanent ostomy. If the ostomy is permanent, malfunctioning or diseased parts are severed, removed, and usually discarded. If the ostomy is temporary, severed parts may still be left in the body. After healing or stabilizing takes place, surgery may reconnect (in medical terminology, reanastomose) the severed parts, so that natural functioning can be reestablished.

Every ostomy is performed for a different reason. This depends on a lot of things, including your condition, your body, physique, and needs. Every ostomy functions in a specific way. This determines how you will take care of it, and what kind of equipment you'll use. Are you ready to explore the main types of ostomies?

COLOSTOMIES

Approximately two-thirds of all ostomy surgeries are colostomies. Because colostomies result from obstruction or cancer-related problems, many colostomy patients are individuals in their fifties or older. The ratio between men and women is approximately the same.

In the colostomy, part of the large intestine is either disconnected or removed. In addition, all or part of the rectum may have to be removed. The colostomy may be performed on any part of the large intestine. This location determines the specific name of the colostomy performed. There are four different types of colostomies, depending on exactly where in the large intestine it is created. Think, for example, about the direction waste moves as it proceeds through your intestines. If the colostomy is in the part of the large intestine where waste matter moves upward, it is called an ascending colostomy. If the colostomy is made in the part of the colon that goes across the body, it's called a transverse colostomy. If the surgery is in the part of the colon that goes back down towards the rectum, it's called a descending colostomy. If it occurs in the part connecting the descending colon with the rectum, it's called a sigmoid colostomy. Descending and sigmoid colostomies are the most common types.

What, Exactly, Is Done?

An artificial opening is surgically created in the abdominal wall. The location of the stoma usually depends on what part of the colon is affected. Since most colostomies are descending colostomies, the opening is usually placed on the lower left side of the abdomen, slightly above the hip bone. Most of the colon is functioning, and only the last portion is disconnected or removed. The end of the healthy length of the large intestine is then brought to the opening on the abdominal wall and sewn. The stoma itself usually protrudes anywhere from a quarter to a half an inch away from the abdominal wall, rather than being totally flat.

Double Barrel or Loop Colostomies

In most cases, when the colostomy is permanent, the rectum and anus are removed. If it is hoped that the colostomy will be temporary, as is frequently the case in ascending or transverse colostomies, the balance of the colon is usually not removed. The colostomy may have been necessary to give a "resting period" to the remaining length of intestine. Frequently, one of two special types of colostomies may be performed: a double barrel or loop colostomy. Both procedures are usually temporary, although they may be permanent. Two stomas are created. One discharges waste; the other one, only a little mucous. In fact, the other stoma may not discharge anything. It sometimes shrivels up and becomes somewhat less noticeable. In the double barrel (or divided) colostomy, the colon is actually severed. Each end is brought to the abdominal wall, forming a stoma. The two stomas are usually right next to each other. Sometimes a segment of the intestine will be removed as well. In such cases, the two stomas, the active one and the "mucous one," will not be located as closely to each other.

In the loop colostomy, the colon is not cut all the way through. Rather, one side of it is sliced. At that point, the intestine is folded all the way back, with both new openings brought to the surface. Because it has not been completely severed, the non-functioning end does not shrivel up. Usually there will be a small discharge of mucous.

In both methods, once healing has taken place (maybe over several months or a year) and it is determined that the entire colon can function once again, it is a fairly simple procedure to reconnect the cut ends.

The loop colostomy is usually preferable to the double barrel colostomy. Why? Once healing has taken place, it is easier to reconnect partly severed segments than totally severed segments. The difficulty with the loop colostomy, however, is that the stoma is usually very large. An entire loop of colon must be brought out through the abdominal wall to form the double opening. Something must be inserted to hold the colon to the inside of the abdominal wall until the inside incision heals. This is usually some type of rod or plastic apparatus. It will hold the intestine snugly against the abdominal wall and should usually remain in place for several days after surgery. Some people have reported that, with the size of the loop colostomy and its unusual shape, it may be more difficult to get a proper fit of an appliance used to collect waste. This, however, is not always the case. Your E.T. can help you to get fitted properly.

ILEOSTOMIES

Approximately 20 to 25 percent of ostomies are ileostomies, and these are performed more often in females. Most ileostomates are teens or young adults. An ileostomy is a surgical procedure that usually involves the removal or disconnection of the entire large intestine. The end of the small intestine (the ileum) is brought through the surgically created opening in the abdominal wall and sewn, forming the stoma. In some cases, part of the small intestine may be removed as well. The new end point will then be brought through the abdominal wall to form the stoma.

Occasionally, temporary ileostomies are performed. In such cases, the large intestine is not always removed. Rather, a segment of the healthy small intestine may be constructed into an ileostomy, remaining in place until healing is complete in the diseased intestine below it. At this time, the segments of the intestine are reconnected (reanastomosed). The ileostomy stoma should protrude further than that of the colostomy. In this way, the looser waste can flow into the appliance without leakage. The "nipple" of the ileostomy stoma usually protrudes anywhere from three fourths of an inch to an inch.

More and more, the rectum is being removed along with the large intestine, especially in cases of ulcerative colitis or familial polyposis. Why? When the anus and rectum do remain in place, they no longer function. However, they must be checked periodically to be sure that no additional problems arise. The rectum is actually an extension of the colon. Its removal helps to prevent any further disease or cancer in the remaining portion.

Continent Ileostomies

Although the conventional ileostomy we've just discussed has been successful in improving conditions for thousands of individuals, sometimes alternate procedures are used. One newer technique is called the continent ileostomy, or Kock pouch, developed by the Swedish surgeon Nils Kock in the late 1960's. The colon and rectum are removed. The last segment of the small intestine (ranging from at least several inches up to about 18 inches) is looped to form a pouch (or reservoir) with a valve, inside the abdomen. A segment of the intestine extends from the reservoir to the abdominal wall. The end part forms the stoma. Waste matter can then accumulate in this pouch, within the body, rather than flowing out through the stoma. After a period of time, the reservoir within the abdomen gradually stretches until it can eventually hold at least a pint of waste.

So why is it called a continent ileostomy? Medically, continent means being able to retain waste until an appropriate time for release. For example, someone in a coma who has no ability to control excretion is said to be incontinent. If we do have that control, we are continent. With a continent ileostomy, waste is retained in the reservoir. The valve in the reservoir prohibits the passage of waste material or gas out through the stoma, until a tube (catheter) is inserted. A few times each day, the ostomate inserts a tube to catheterize (or trigger the release of waste in) the reservoir. This procedure is called intubation. The waste drains out through the tube, into either the toilet or a receptacle. If the stool is too thick when the reservoir is catheterized, water may be inserted through the catheter to thin it. The reservoir is usually emptied three to five times a day.

The main advantage of the continent ileostomy is that you don't have to wear an appliance. Usually, all you have to wear is a patch or bandage over your stoma for protection. As a result, the stoma doesn't need to protrude the usual three-quarters of an inch to an inch, as in conventional ileostomies. The stoma is still necessary for drainage, but it doesn't work nearly as often as stomas through which waste passes regularly. Because of this, the continent ileostomy stoma can be placed on your abdomen in a more desirable place. Since appliances are not required, more fashionable clothing (including skimpier bathing suits) may be worn if your figure is right!

If continent ileostomies are so great, then why aren't all ileostomies of this type? Why don't individuals with conventional ileostomies have surgery to change to the internal continent ileostomy? There are three reasons. First, although some may decide to convert from one to the other through new surgery, others may feel that they have grown accustomed to what they've got. Therefore, they have chosen not to convert. Second, and even more important, continent ileostomies are not advised for all ileostomates. In order for the continent ileostomy to be successful, the pouch or reservoir must remain disease-free. Evidence indicates that Crohn's disease may continue to attack portions of intestine that remain in the body. Therefore, because the small intestine is used to form the reservoir, Crohn's may affect the pouch or valve controlling the flow of waste after surgery. If you have Crohn's disease, therefore, you really shouldn't have a continent ileostomy. But if you've suffered from ulcerative colitis or familial polyposis, your surgeon may suggest the continent ileostomy. Although many surgeries for continent ileostomies are successful, some may not be, due to a variety of complications. As a result, appliances may have to be worn even with the continent ileostomy, or surgery may be necessary to return to a conventional ileostomy.

What are the complications that can cause a failure of continent ileostomy surgery? Your pouch may leak or there might be a malfunction in the valve (the valve could slip or not be able to prevent stool and gas from exiting the body). These are two of the more common complications. Other problems include difficulties with intubation, or the formation of fistulae or scar tissue within the pouch of the intestines. In some cases, another operation (maybe even more than one) may be necessary to correct the problems.

Approximately half of today's continent ileostomies are being done as original surgeries. The other half are revisions of the conventional ileostomies.

Ileorectal Anastomosis

The ileorectal anastomosis procedure is another alternative to the conventional ileostomy. In this procedure the surgeon, rather than bringing the small intestine to the abdominal wall in a stoma, connects the small intestine directly to the rectum. In this way, feces can be eliminated directly from the rectum, and no stoma is needed. Although this may sound more desirable than other ileostomy procedures, it has its problems. One concern is that of a higher risk of rectal cancer. It is also possible for ulcerative colitis to recur (if this was the cause of surgery in the first place). Why? In order for the procedure to be successful, at least a small amount of mucous membrane from the rectum must remain intact. The intestine is connected to this segment. But proper treatment of ulcerative colitis or familial polyposis requires that no mucous membrane whatsoever be left behind. So these conditions probably wouldn't be considered suitable for the ileorectal anastamosis procedure. However, if the rectum is not affected by the surgery-causing illness, (for example, if Crohn's disease has not affected the rectum), then this procedure may be considered.

Endo-Rectal Ileal Pull-Through

Yet another alternative to the conventional ileostomy is the "endo-rectal ileal pull-through." In this case, instead of having the small intestine connected to the mucous membrane of the rectum, the ileum is pulled through the rectum and attached to its end. The problem with this procedure is that the "signals" for defecation will continue. Because of the looser consistency of waste matter, you'll become a "short-distance runner," feeling this need many times a day! This will place added stress on your sphincter muscles, besides being a pain in the neck. With proper training, however, it might be possible to "teach" your anal muscles how to handle this more frequent, looser flow of waste. Is this procedure for you? Maybe, but probably not if you've been diagnosed with Crohn's disease. Once again, because of the possibility of recurring diseases in the new rectal area, your surgeon would most likely reject this type of technique.

Anything Else Under the Abdomen?

This section would not be complete without mentioning that more efficient alternatives to the ones described above are always being probed by research. One such method, still in the investigative stage, is a procedure in which an ileal reservoir is created near the place where the ileum is connected (anastomosed) to the anus. What will they think of next? Stay tuned.

UROSTOMIES

The third main category of ostomies we will discuss, including about 10 to 15 percent of all ostomy surgeries, is the urostomy. Urostomates range in age from infancy to the elderly, although almost one fourth of all urostomies occur in young children. In children, urostomies are usually necessary treatment for congenital birth defects. In adults, spinal cord injuries or cancer are the usual causes of urostomies.

Urostomies are also known as urinary diversions because they divert the flow of urine away from disease or damage in the kidneys, bladder, urethra, or ureters. The diverted urine flows into a passageway leading to the stoma in the abdominal wall. Because urine always remains in liquid form, being discharged almost continuously, appliances must be worn at all times.

There are a few different types of urinary diversions. The specific name of the urostomy is determined by where in the urinary tract the surgery occurs and how it is performed.

Ileal Conduit

The ileal conduit, originally developed in 1950, has become the most common type of urostomy. Now don't be confused. The ileal conduit is not an ileostomy, even though it contains the word "ileal." Rather, part of the small intestine (ileal) is used as the tube transporting urine to the stoma. How? A short segment of the small intestine, usually four to eight inches long, is removed from the rest of the small intestine (which is then reconnected). One end of the new segment is closed. The narrow tubes (the ureters) that carry urine away from the kidneys are inserted inside this ileum tube. The segment is then connected to the abdominal wall, forming the stoma, and acts as a passageway, or conduit, for urine. As with ileostomies, the nipple of the stoma should protrude three quarters of an inch to an inch. In this way, the urine can easily flow into the appliance collecting it, with less chance of leakage. The conduit does not have any storage capacity. Therefore, it only serves as a passageway, and urine is almost continuously flowing out of the stoma.

Colonic Conduit

Occasionally, problems arise in using pieces of the ileum as the passageways of urine. One possible solution is using a portion of the colon instead. That's where the name colonic conduit comes from. The surgery is done the same way as with the ileal conduit: a segment of the colon is removed, one end is closed, the other end is attached to the abdominal wall, forming the stoma, and the ureters are both inserted into it. The remaining parts of the colon are reconnected. One advantage of the colonic conduit is that, because the diameter is larger than that of the ileal conduit, there is less chance of stoma-related complications.

Other Forms of Urostomies

Another type of urostomy is the ureterostomy. The narrow tubes from the kidneys, the ureters, are brought directly through the abdominal wall, forming small but efficient stomas. This is an alternative to inserting the ureters in another conduit. Depending upon the condition of the ureters, your surgeon will determine if either or both should be brought to the abdominal wall. One problem with ureterostomies is that the ureters may narrow or constrict, restricting the flow of urine. This can be dangerous. Infection can result from the backing up of urine in the kidney. Therefore, it is necessary for you to carefully monitor the urine flow, and to notice any reduction in output that may indicate a problem.

A vesicostomy brings the bladder itself directly to the abdominal wall. A surgical opening is made so that urine can flow directly from the bladder to the outside. No tubes are used. The placement of the vesicostomy on the bladder determines whether the bladder will be able to store urine (so that the bladder can be drained using a catheter), or whether no storage is possible (with urine flowing constantly).

Whereas the vesicostomy brings the bladder to the abdominal wall, the pyelostomy brings the kidney directly to the flank. As with ileal or colonic conduits or ureterostomies, this totally bypasses the bladder, but no tubes are used. A big problem with this procedure is that it is hard to get an appliance to fit the opening created by such a stoma. Another concern is that extreme caution must be used to prevent any urine that has been diverted out of the body from flowing back into the kidney.

A nephrostomy involves inserting a tube from outside the abdominal wall directly into the kidney to drain the urine. There is a higher risk of infection in this procedure and it is usually, if not always, done as a temporary procedure.

Finally, an older procedure that isn't done as much anymore is the ureterosigmoidostomy. Here the urine is diverted directly into the sigmoid colon. In other words, urine leaves the body through the anal sphincter. This procedure was more common earlier in the twentieth century. Kidney infection, developing from bacterial growth in the colon, is just one example of the risks of this procedure.

4

Surgery—Before and After

If you are reading this book, but have not yet had your ostomy surgery, there are probably some very important things on your mind. (Even if you have had your surgery, the questions don't stop!) Not only will you be concerned with your future health, but you'll also be concerned with your future activities and relationships. As you read through this book, you will see that most of your possible concerns are handled in complete detail, in order to provide you with some reassurances. You'll see that there *is* "life after surgery"!

BEFORE. . . .

Want to hear a shocker? Did you know that, according to a recent study, over one third of all ostomates received no prior preparation for this surgery? Many doctors simply didn't take the time. Maybe they thought someone else would explain what was going to happen.

Once you've heard those dreaded words that you're going to need surgery, then what? For most of you, if you've had advance notice of your impending surgery, you'll have the unpleasantness of anticipating the "event." Some of you may not have much, if any, warning. You may need surgery because of a life-threatening condition. This may come about so quickly that there is no anticipation at all. An auto accident, an injury, or some other circumstance may thrust you into the operating room. In this case, you are only aware of your ostomy surgery after it's a "fait accompli." If that's the case, the first part of this chapter does not apply to you as much.

The time of anticipation before surgery can be among the most difficult times ever experienced. The longer the waiting period before your surgery, the more anxiety you may build up. If you've been ill for a while, for example, your doctors may have told you that if you didn't get better with other treatment, ostomy surgery might be necessary. So this may have been in the back of your mind for a long time. Does that mean you're always upset about it? No. What if you've been experiencing a lot of discomfort, and your physicians have told you that it will go away after surgery? It probably won't be as undesirable an alternative!

You can help yourself feel better during this nail-biting time. Be sure to ask lots of questions. You *are* entitled to know what's going to happen, and why. Make sure that all the questions you can think of are answered before surgery. The exceptions, of course, are those questions that cannot be answered! Even then, it's reassuring to know that a professional recognizes your apprehensions. What questions should you ask? Ask about the reasons for your ostomy surgery. Be assured that, for the most part, surgery is not performed unless there is a real necessity. But you can certainly question why it's necessary. In some cases, you may anticipate the need for surgery even before you've been told. But what if the surgery diagnosis comes as a surprise? You may have a harder time dealing with this. Ask other questions as well, including where the stoma will be, how your intestines will function, and so on. Ask what your convalescence will be like. Find out who will be helping you. This group will include enterostomal therapists (E.T.'s), who are specialists in helping ostomates.

Contact your local chapter of the United Ostomy Association or a similar group. Remember: the more you prepare yourself, the better everything will be. To quote yet another research study (no, that's not all I do with my time!), individuals who are more adequately prepared prior to surgery do better in surgery and, even more importantly, after. Therefore, it is important for you to learn as much as you can beforehand. Knowledge can improve your attitude. You want to know that you can communicate with the professionals responsible for your care.

If you're afraid of your surgery or of being in the hospital, there may be some pre-surgical activities that are anxiety-provoking for you. For example, the tests and extensive examinations that must be done before surgery may not be your idea of a good time. Other pre-surgical procedures, including enemas (when appropriate), shaving (where appropriate), and pre-surgical medications, aren't thrilling either.

.... AND AFTER

Not too many people enjoy the time following surgery when they're recovering from the effects of general anesthesia. The anesthetic is important in creating the deep unconsciousness necessary for painless (and successful) surgery. After surgery, however, you may experience some uncomfortable side effects. This will pass.

After surgery, you'll spend some time in the recovery room. There you will be closely checked for any post-surgical complications. Oxygen will be provided, not because there is a problem, but because it will help to clear out your lungs and make breathing easier. Coughing is necessary to clear the airsacs.

Not too long after surgery (it may seem like ten minutes!) you'll be instructed to get out of bed and walk. (Why does this always seem like a command, not a request? And why does it always seem to come from a nurse who looks like she'll throw you out of bed if you don't comply?) You may not be too eager to do this, but it's really necessary for both your circulation as well as your breathing.

How do you like having tubes sticking out all over your body? Not too wonderful! The IV tube you probably expected. But what about the tube going through your nose and down into your stomach? This is used to remove any digestive secretions, since there will be no food in the stomach for them to work on. Another tube may also be necessary for bladder catheterization. Tubes don't last forever, though. It won't be long until they're gone (but not forgotten!).

One of the hardest parts of coping with an ostomy is seeing the incision and your stoma for the first time. Many ostomates have reacted with shock, anxiety, disbelief, or utter despair upon seeing their "rosebuds" for the first time. Because of this, prior preparation usually helps. Speak to your physician, E.T.'s, or other ostomates, look at diagrams, and so on. All of this can help you to prepare for the first review of the battlefield.

THE VISITORS PROGRAM

So you've had ostomy surgery. You probably have plenty of questions, and you're probably experiencing a whole range of unpleasant emotional reactions. What do you do? Your physicians won't have enough time, other professionals may not always be available, and your family and friends will be having their own difficulties. A "visitor" can be a big help. The Visitors Program was established by the United Ostomy Association (UOA). Although it's not a unique concept, this effective program arranges for individuals who have had ostomy surgery in the past to voluntarily visit new ostomates. During these visits, they can answer many of your questions. In addition, they will demonstrate (by example!) that individuals with ostomies can function. In many cases, it's almost impossible to tell that they have had surgery or are wearing appliances. For example, a frequent first reaction of new ostomates when visited by a stylishly dressed "visitor" is, "These people can't be ostomates. They're wearing 'normal' clothes!" Soon they are pleasantly surprised to find out that they were wrong.

Initially, were you unwilling to talk about your surgery? Did you try to deny it? Push it away? Depression may be one reason for this. In some of these cases, visitors from the UOA may be requested by family or by professionals. Visitors will understand if you do not want to talk about the surgery at first. It may take a little time to draw out your feelings. But visitors have had experience and training in dealing with these situations. You will learn that you should not be embarrassed to discuss it. Talking about it doesn't mean you're going to walk around and show everybody your stoma, but you can discuss what has happened. This is a start on your road to acceptance.

If your initial reaction to your visitor was negative, this is understandable. If you were trying to push the topic away, you can understand why you did not want someone to come in and bring it up. However, as you start conversing and learning more, you'll begin to look forward to these visits. They'll help you to adjust to your new body image and to your new method of bowel control. Morale can be vastly improved by talking to somebody who has had the same experience.

By the way, if you had your surgery a while ago, you can be a big help! Talk to other "ostomates-to-be." Share experiences. Let them know how you felt, but always emphasize the fact that you're adjusting more and more each day.

A FINAL HELPFUL POST-SURGICAL NOTE

As long as we're talking about people who can be of tremendous comfort and support after your surgery, this chapter would not be complete without mentioning the enterostomal therapist. Enterostomal therapists (E.T.'s) are a group of dedicated nurses, with specialized training in working with ostomates. In this book I often mention the advantages of consulting an E.T. But what happens if you don't know where to find one? Or what if there aren't any in your local hospital? You still have a couple of choices. You could contact the International Association for Enterostomal Therapy (see the address in Appendix) for names of the nearest E.T.'s, or mention the problem to your physician, nurse, or ostomy chapter representative.

So don't be concerned about reaching out. You can always find warm, caring people who are eager to help.

5

Appliances and Equipment

This chapter doesn't focus on refrigerators, dishwashers, washers, or dryers. Waste compactors aren't addressed, either, but you're getting closer! Once you have ostomy surgery, there must be a new way to collect the waste material expelled from your body, since surgery has eliminated the toilet as the "receptacle of choice." Wearing an "appliance," also called a pouch or some other names (be nice!), is the main method used. It is worn over the stoma, allowing the waste material to go directly into it. The appliance is, therefore, necessary for collecting waste as well as avoiding embarrassment, due to the staining and ruining of clothing (and reputation).

Not all ostomates need to wear appliances. The type of surgery determines whether or not an appliance is required. For example, urostomy surgery almost always requires a pouch, but colostomy surgery may not. A special management technique, irrigation, may eliminate the need for an appliance. Ileostomy surgery may not require an appliance if a continent ileostomy is created. Remember that, in a continent ileostomy, a reservoir is formed inside the body by using a portion of the small intestine. Waste material accumulates there and is drained using intubation (a catheter procedure). Appliances aren't necessary.

HISTORY OF APPLIANCES

Not too long ago, you didn't have much choice! There were very few appliances to choose from. Children with ostomies had even more difficulty finding appliances that would meet their needs. As recently as the late

1940's, there was such a small variety of appliances available that those who did have ostomy surgery didn't even want to wear them. Instead, they used dressings or bulky pads.

But let's go back even further and do some historical "appliance watching." In 1795, a French surgeon designed a small leather bag (not a purse!), which could probably be considered one of the first colostomy appliances. But this didn't start the ball rolling. Why? Ostomy surgery was not done frequently until the middle of the twentieth century. With an increase in ostomy surgery, there was more and more variety in appliances. Another why? Patient demand! As more and more people had ostomy surgery, they became more vocal in their need for light-weight appliances. They didn't want the bulky inconvenience of pads and dressings. In addition, ostomates wanted new appliances to prevent embarrassing odors. Spillage was another concern. So ostomates demanded leak-proof, spill-proof appliances to increase their feelings of security.

The demands were heard. Appliance companies grew and began to fashion the necessary equipment out of plastic. Plastic satisfied many needs. New appliances were light-weight, easily adaptable, and partially controlled odor and leakage problems. Where did such a variety of new appliances come from? Surgical supply houses or hospital supply companies, recognizing the need for appliances because of the growing number of ostomates, were most active. But that's not all. The ostomates themselves got into the act. Frustrated ostomates, wanting more appropriate equipment, developed far better devices than were available. Many designed their own appliances because they simply refused to wear the old-fashioned, wired pouches. These did not have proper openings, and were unreliable in collecting waste. They were difficult to dispose of, and could not be easily attached to the skin. This contributed to leakage. Skin irritation (and embarrassment) resulted. If that wasn't enough, old appliances were uncomfortable and ostomates could only wear loose fitting, unfashionable clothing.

So new appliance styles were born out of desperation. But where else did ideas for new devices come from? Frequently, they came from the ostomates' "professional representatives," enterostomal therapists. These specialists play a very important role in updating all ostomy-related equipment. They are instrumental in recommending a specific type of device (or, in some cases, even designing it!) They test and evaluate new products before they even become available for consumers.

Much progress has been made in developing modern, efficient appliances. The future will probably see even more advances, with the rise of new and even more competent equipment. Yet, the variety available to ostomates today is certainly far superior to the way it used to be. There are devices that can be used either immediately or easily modified to suit your ostomy needs, including stoma location and size, as well as your physical and emotional needs. Your enterostomal therapist will generally make appropriate recommendations.

TYPES OF APPLIANCES

Before we begin discussing appliances, adhesives, and all those other goodies, you must remember something. Many factors determine what you're going to use. This chapter only provides you with some general information about what's available. You should work together with your physician, nurse, or enterostomal therapist (E.T.) to decide what's best for you.

Knowing what to use is easy during the first few weeks after surgery. You'll have to wait for post-surgical swelling to go down, and for your stoma to become stable in size. During that short period of time, you'll wear temporary appliances. You'll usually start with transparent pouches, which are affixed to the skin directly following surgery. Because they are transparent, enterostomal therapists, physicians, nurses, or other helping professionals can see that your stoma is functioning properly and is in good condition.

Appliances come in many different sizes, shapes, and colors, and are made out of different materials. The type of appliances you'll be most comfortable wearing depends on a number of variables. These include the size and shape of your stoma, the type of surgery you've had, your age and sex, your desires (your personality may enter the picture here), and your financial condition.

When will you start thinking about this? Not for awhile. A new ostomate rarely thinks about what type of appliances to use. Your E.T.

will help to fit you with the correct equipment. After some time has passed (sometimes many months), you may hear about an appliance you'd like to try. Have confidence in your E.T.'s appraisal of your needs, and discuss it.

You may ultimately wear different appliances than the types you started with. Tastes change, feelings change, abilities change, symptoms change, skin conditions change, and this is no "small change!" As a matter of fact, you may wear different appliances under different circumstances. For example, you might wear a different appliance for exercise than you would when you sleep. You might also wear a different appliance when you travel than when you work.

Permanent vs. Temporary Appliances

There are two basic types of appliances. The reusable or permanent appliance is cleaned out, washed, dried, and then used again. They can be cleaned repeatedly, and are usually made of odor-proof material so that odors are kept inside (and away from embarrassment). Even if you use permanent appliances, you'll probably keep extras on hand so you can rotate them between uses. In this way, they'll be completely dry before their next use. You'll probably even want to have a few disposables on hand in case of an emergency.

Disposable appliances are usually thrown out after one use. That use can last up to about a week, but these appliances cannot be cleaned and reused. Disposable appliances, also called single use or expendable appliances, have one big advantage: it's a lot easier to just throw them away instead of cleaning them out and making sure that they are sanitary. The disadvantage is that costs are higher. You must purchase more, since you keep throwing them away. Your needs and other practical issues will determine the kind of appliances to select.

Children may not have as much of a choice. Children usually have to change their appliances more frequently. Because of this, it may be smart for them to wear permanent appliances. On the other hand, children may prefer lightweight, plastic, disposable pouches. Chance of leakage can be reduced by proper use of skin sealants, stomahesives, or other preventives. More about that later.

One-Piece vs. Two-Piece Appliances

Another way of categorizing appliances is to talk about one-piece and two-piece appliances. The one-piece appliance attaches directly to the skin, using an adhesive or sealant. In addition to the adhesive, you might use tape to be sure your pouch is securely attached to the skin. The one-piece pouch is usually emptied from the bottom when it is from one-third to one-half full.

In two-piece appliances, one piece is called the face plate; the other, the pouch. The face plate is attached to the skin, similar to the way the one-piece appliance is attached. A type of ostomy cement (not Krazy Glue!) is usually used, and allowed to dry thoroughly before the pouch is attached. The face plate usually remains in place for up to a week. It's not a permanent addition to the body. Two-piece appliances may be used by ostomates who have difficulty using one-piece devices. For example, it may be advisable if excessive removal and replacement irritates your skin. You don't need to use permanent appliances if you're using permanent face plates. You can attach temporary or disposable appliances to the face plate. Regardless of whether the appliance is a one or two-piece device, it can be worn up to seven days. A protective skin barrier should be worn under the pouch and around the stoma.

The Receptacle

The pouch itself usually comes with either an open end or a closed end. The open-ended pouch is drainable and can be either reusable or disposable. The pouch usually has some kind of closure (a clip or tie) at the end (what good would it be otherwise?), so that it will remain securely fastened and closed until you're ready to empty it. An open-ended urinary appliance may have a valve to allow easy drainage. At the same time, it will provide adequate protection against leakage when the valve is closed.

Open-ended pouches are used by ileostomates or urostomates. Closed-end devices require the removal of your pouch many times a day. Open-ended pouches, therefore, make life easier.

The closed-end pouch is more commonly used by the colostomate because waste material is more firm. You're also less likely to be concerned about drainage. You'll probably just discard the whole thing. But you can also use open-ended pouches, especially if your colostomy is located in a place where the feces will not be as firm. The looser the consistency of the waste material, the more likely that you'll use the same type of appliance as an ileostomate.

How About Size?

You might decide to wear smaller pouches during the day, since you may be changing or draining them anyway. On the other hand, you may use larger ones at night so you can have a more comfortable sleep without worrying about spillage, overflow, leakage, or discomfort. Smaller pouches are used by athletes or by individuals who like to wear skimpy clothing, such as bathing suits.

The size of the appliance you'll use also depends on your age. Obviously, smaller appliances are going to be used with children. But they can't be *too* small, since children can't store as much in their bodies. Waste material will flow quickly into the appliance, and require very frequent emptying if the appliance is too small.

What Else?

Besides coming in many sizes and shapes, appliances may also come in many colors and be made out of different materials. The type of material you select may depend on your skin. If you sweat easily, plastic may not be the best material, since it may be uncomfortable. Colors are usually a determining factor only if you really get a kick out of that kind of thing! How many people will see them, anyhow? Then again, how many people see your underwear, and look at the variety here!

The material used may vary according to the type of ostomy. The material used for appliances in urostomies is usually latex or light-weight vinyl, or opaque or transparent plastic. Such material is usually most resistant to the chemical action of urine. Urine does not usually present the same type of odor problems as feces. Therefore, the material used in making appliances for ileostomies and colostomies must be odor-proof. Vinyl or synthetic rubber is usually best for this. Manufacturers will always state specifications about the appliances they produce, including whether they are odor-proof, the type of material, and how long they should last.

WHAT IF YOU DON'T NEED AN APPLIANCE?

Irrigating colostomates and continent ileostomates are among those of you who may not need appliances. You might prefer to use a pad, patch, bandage, or dressing of some type. This would cover the opening, and protect your clothing from the leakage of waste matter or mucous. Some irrigators choose to wear a "security" pouch for added protection.

ADHESIVES TO GET "STUCK ON"

The use of the proper adhesive is almost as important as the appliance itself. If you do not have confidence in your adhesive, you may be concerned that the appliance will not remain firmly and securely in place. If so, watch out for leakage!

Adhesives should be water-resistant. They should adhere firmly to the skin. Special adhesives must be used for urostomates, so that urine doesn't break down their holding power. Adhesives must also be resistant to perspiration. During the summer, you certainly don't want your appliance to fall off because the adhesive has melted!

The adhesive that will work best with your appliance depends on the type of appliance, your skin sensitivity, and other variables. If you're using a permanent face plate, you'll want your adhesive to be a type of long-lasting cement. If a disposable appliance is used, the adhesive must still help it to stay securely in place until it needs to be changed. Since this may be up to seven days, you might want to reinforce the adhesive with tape. Materials such as stoma adhesives are used frequently in order to meet many ostomy management needs. You may have to experiment with adhesives in order to determine what's best for you. What happens if your skin is so sensitive that any adhesive irritates you? In this case, a non-irritating type of tape may have to be used. If that doesn't work, check with your E.T. for other options.

SKIN BARRIERS

Whenever the skin around the stoma is exposed, it's always a good idea to use a skin barrier. This skin barrier, usually applied to the area between the stoma itself and the face plate, protects the skin from irritation that might result if there was contact with the waste material. The skin barrier is usually used as the adhesive when the appliance is put on. When the appliance is changed, it can be gently washed off, and the skin area cleansed. Cleaning also prevents a build-up of the barrier that you use.

There are a number of different substances that may be used as skin protection. For example, stomahesives, powders, pastes, sprays, or even pliable and moldable sheets, which can be made of plastic or other materials. More solid substances may also be used, with backing. These backings may be of plastic, or may have a mesh-like backing. It is important that all skin barriers, especially those with backings, be cut and shaped carefully. In this way, they'll provide the best possible protection without damaging your stoma.

Skin barriers have been recognized, used, and available for more than ten years. Although they have added greatly to the comfort of wearing appliances, they can also create difficulties if not used properly. Some skin barriers might even cause skin irritation instead of protecting you from it. Make sure this doesn't happen. How? Try a modified test. To do this, select a small area of skin in an inconspicuous place. Apply the skin barrier to see if there is any kind of reaction within 48 hours. If redness, swelling, burning, or itching occurs, don't use this skin barrier! If, after 48 hours, there is no noticeable reaction, the skin barrier is probably safe for you to use.

Some skin barriers can be used even after skin irritation has developed. These are designed not only to protect the skin, but also to promote healing of the irritated skin. For this reason, they usually contain treatment medications. Should skin barriers be used by every ostomate? Opinions differ, and each individual case is different.

What's the best way to determine how to use skin barriers? There are two important steps. First, consult a professional, such as an E.T. You'll get expert advice as to what barriers might be best for your particular situation. Second, be sure to follow the manufacturer's instructions for any skin barrier you decide to try. As with appliances, you'll probably have to experiment in order to find the best skin barrier for you.

DEODORANTS

All ostomates are concerned about odor. As a matter of fact, it's such a big worry that we'll cover it in greater detail later on. But let's touch on the subject briefly here, since we're talking about useful equipment. Fortunately, in recent years, appliances have either contained deodorants or could be deodorized. This has reduced the chances of embarrassing odor. Many appliances are now made of very effective, odor-proof material. This has not totally eliminated concern about odor, however. Gas build-up can be a problem, and must be released. Otherwise, the consequences can be explosive! In order for gas to be released without embarrassing odor, the use of charcoal or other deodorizing agents in the release valve might be helpful.

Deodorizers used during appliance cleaning usually come in liquid form. They generally do a good job of ridding the appliance of lingering odor. These can deodorize the appliance during cleaning or even during normal wear. Any other ideas? Many ostomates take certain substances by mouth, which can help to neutralize many odor problems. Certain natural foods (such as parsley), mouth washes, or oral deodorizers (such as Binaca), may be helpful.

FACE PLATES

If you've chosen to wear a two-piece appliance, your face plate has taken on very important significance. The size and shape of this face plate, as well as the way you attach it to your body, are very important. Body contour and stoma placement are important factors in choosing the right face plate. Work with your E.T. This will help assure you of proper fitting.

There are several standard openings for face plates. This can make it easy to fit, unless your stoma is irregularly shaped. If it is, you might take a measurement of the stoma and send it to the manufacturer. Most manufacturers will be more than happy to sell you a properly-fitted face plate.

You want to have as much mobility as you can, without any restrictions. Therefore, the face plate should be of a light material (such as plastic), if possible. Some face plates are moldable. This will make it easier for you to attach it securely to your body. Each person's body contour is different. You'll feel a lot better knowing that your plate securely adheres to your own body contour. The edges of your face plate should be smooth, as well. Can you guess why? Well, you certainly don't want another source of irritation, nor do you want to take the chance of cutting your stoma.

Even face plates that are considered permanent should usually be changed. Why? Cleaning time! It's recommended that you do this approximately once a week. You may want to change and clean your face plate more often if it's not attached as securely, if there has been any accumulation of urine or feces under it, or if any leakage or skin irritation problems occur.

OTHER NECESSARY EQUIPMENT

What other equipment might be helpful? How about appliance covers? These goodies, usually made of a soft, washable fabric, tend to fit appliances the way fitted sheets cover your mattress. The material will absorb perspiration, preventing skin irritation. The soft fabric helps to make your appliance as comfortable as possible, especially in warm weather. Covers may also be colorful. Can you imagine how this can help your intimate interpersonal relationships? On the other hand, maybe you don't want to wear those things! They may only add to the appliance's bulk. You may feel it is more noticeable under your clothing. The decision is up to you.

These next two paragraphs will really give you a belt! Some ostomates do wear belts for added support. Although these can make appliances a little more comfortable as they fill up, they will not prevent leaking. A disadvantage of using a belt is that it's something else to take care of. If you do decide to use them, make sure they're not too tight. That can cause damage to the skin. You may choose to wear belts only at night, when traveling, or at other specific times, to provide added security. If you choose to wear them, you'll decide the most appropriate times.

Belts come in a variety of different shapes, and are made of a number of different materials. Different fasteners (such as buckles, hooks, or velcro) may be used. The belt is usually connected to the appliance itself, so that it won't slip off. However, because the belt is affixed to the appliance, problems may occur if it is too loose or too tight. This may prevent the appliance from moving in a natural way as it fills or as your body moves.

Finally, you might decide you want to use tape from time to time. Tape can provide added security. It will help to keep the appliance securely attached to your skin. Most tapes are waterproof, flexible, and usually safe for the skin. However, if your skin is sensitive, there are non-allergenic tapes that may be used. Old-fashioned adhesive tapes are not the best choice. Why not? Tape has to be changed frequently. Adhesive tapes are sticky, and therefore hard to remove. This can cause skin irritation. Paper tapes similar to the non-allergenic tapes can be good for this purpose.

A FITTING CONCLUSION

There are many different ways to care for your stoma, and there's a variety of appliances and other equipment available. Don't feel restricted. You might even want to be more creative and fashion your own appliances, using whatever materials are appropriate for your needs. There is such an increasing assortment of ostomy appliances and equipment, however, that unless you really like to be inventive, this should not be necessary.

Who do you ask? It is extremely helpful to speak with your enterostomal therapist. Although nurses, physicians, or other individuals who have gone through this may have some ideas, your E.T. has been trained to help you quickly and efficiently. Why waste time experimenting when you can get everything together rapidly?

PART II

Your Emotions

6

Coping with your Emotions — An Introduction

Are you happy about having an ostomy? Now don't gag on that question! Each person's emotional response to ostomy surgery is different. Even your own emotional reactions will vary from time to time. The more severe your reactions, the more they interfere with your ability to cope.

Your emotional reactions to an ostomy may start even before surgery. They may begin at the time of diagnosis. You may have heard about the experiences of other ostomates. You may have read things that frighten you. It is unlikely, however, that your emotional reactions at this time will match the intensity of those following surgery, when you first get a view of your new addition.

The emotional reactions to ostomy surgery are not always rational. As a matter of fact, in many cases they are completely irrational.

MOURNING YOUR LOSS

Elizabeth Kubler-Ross, in her classic book *On Death And Dying*, outlined the stages that the bereaved or terminally ill person has to work through, starting with shock and denial, and ending with adjustment and acceptance. In a way, the ostomate also has to work through these stages. Why? It's not that you're dying. Rather, don't you feel the loss of your body part or the loss of body functioning? You need to go through the stages of "mourning," instead of suppressing the emotional reactions to ostomy surgery. In this way, the intensity of these emotions will diminish. You'll then be able to more readily accept what has happened, and get on with the rest of your life. More on this in the *Grief* section of the chapter, *Other Emotions*.

YOUR SELF-ESTEEM

Have you experienced a loss of self-esteem? Do you feel that you like
yourself less? Feelings of confidence that have developed to a self-accepting
level may be quickly shattered by the loss of bowel control. This loss can
have a very unpleasant effect on you. You won't feel or behave like yourself. You'll want to deal with this in order to return to effective, efficient
functioning.

FACTORS SHAPING YOUR EMOTIONAL REACTIONS

Several factors may play a role in determining how you react emotionally
to having an ostomy. Keep in mind, though, that no one can predict how
a person will react at any time. There are too many things involved. How
did you handle problems before the need for surgery was diagnosed? What
was your general coping style? Were you calm or nervous? Were you per-
sistent or did you give up easily? Your style of handling life's everyday
problems gives an indication of how you will cope with your ostomy. Are
you successful in coping with stress? Ostomy-related stress may depend on
how fast your problems developed, the cause of surgery, and what the
prognosis is for your condition, among other factors. Your age has a bearing on how you respond emotionally. Also, your general physical health
prior to surgery plays a role in determining your coping ability. In many
cases, your emotional reactions are a reflection of the reactions of significant others in your life. If family members or friends are anxious about
what's happening, this may help to shape your own reactions.

WHICH EMOTIONAL REACTIONS?

Are you furious that an operation like this was necessary? Are you angry
because life will have to be changed as far as waste elimination is concerned? Are you depressed when you compare the present with the way
things were? Are you afraid of not being able to cope? Do you fear a bleak,
if not hopeless, future? Are you afraid because a part of your body was removed, or a new opening added? The removal of certain parts of the body

due to malfunction can be upsetting. Further upset occurs when these changes involve the organs of elimination. This is probably because they are the most private parts of your body. If removed or disconnected, your emotional reaction may be more pronounced.

Some of the most common emotional reactions to having an ostomy are depression, fear, guilt, and anger. Because of the importance of coping with these emotions, a separate chapter has been devoted to each of them, as well as to others, in this section of the book.

HELPING TO MANAGE EMOTIONAL REACTIONS

In the past, adjusting to an ostomy took a long time. More recently, through therapeutic interventions, groups, the wisdom of E.T.'s, and other techniques, the amount of time necessary for adjustment has significantly diminished. Obviously, emotions play an important role in your physical condition. So you certainly want to do the best job possible to control these reactions. How? Let's discuss some of the more important ways.

Medical Management

Make sure you're getting the best possible medical care. You'll want to establish a good working relationship with your physician and E.T. This involves seeing a professional who not only has good knowledge of ostomies but is also understanding, available, and sympathetic to your emotional needs. You'll want to be sure that your physician monitors the healing process, your stoma, and your elimination process to make sure that everything is moving along smoothly (what a choice of words!). If you're on medication, your physician must keep track of your dosages, both to use them most effectively and to minimize any side effects.

Groups

Self-help groups, or coping groups, can be very beneficial. You'll see how others handle problems, which may be exactly the same, or at least similar, to yours. These groups are also wonderful for your family, since one of the best ways to be in control of your emotions is to have a supportive family behind you. The groups provide a forum for the exchange of feelings and ideas, as well as suggestions for how to cope better. They'll show you that you're not alone.

Do you ever feel shunned or ignored by others (or do you fear feeling this way)? Do you find your social relationships dwindling? Groups can give you a feeling of belonging. You don't have to feel alone. There are people with whom you share a common bond, because they also live with ostomies.

In groups, you can discuss any topic you like. You may begin to share feelings more openly, as you hear others bringing up subjects you were previously reluctant to bring up yourself. As a result, a feeling of closeness, almost like a family, develops.

The most important reason for belonging to a group, however, is the sharing of ideas designed to help you cope. Methods of coping and techniques for helping yourself feel better are shared; suggestions are offered and follow-ups can improve these even more.

Belonging to a national organization, such as the United Ostomy Association, can also be helpful. Such organizations bring patients and families together, providing beneficial information. They also help to expand public awareness of ostomies. This will help you with your emotions, since the more people there are who understand what's involved with ostomies, the less alone or isolated you'll feel.

By the way, there is no law that emotional reactions have to be shared with others. It is not necessary to talk about them, even though this can be helpful. But these emotional reactions have to be recognized, and worked through. This will bring about progress. The problem with experiencing emotional reactions lies not in the intensity of what is felt, but rather in the ability to handle what is felt and work through it.

Medication

You'll frequently hear about the use of medication to combat depression, anxiety, anger, and other emotional problems. Antianxiety medication can be helpful, as can mood elevators and antidepressants.

Psychological Strategies

Professional intervention may be necessary if your emotional problems are severe and you want to prevent them from getting worse. Having somebody to talk to may be just the thing to help you cope with your emotions.

Are there any strategies you can start using? Yes. Let's discuss some of the best techniques you can use to improve the way you feel.

Humor can be an amusingly effective way to deal with emotions. Whether it is hearing others' jokes, laughing at one's self, or creating one's own jokes, humor can be a very relaxing way of dealing with a troublesome situation. Basically, humor works in three ways. First of all, it reduces anxiety. Laughing is a great way to release tension. Secondly, it can serve as a distraction from what is bothering you. When you are involved in a humorous situation, you can feel a lot better. If you think back to a time when you were depressed or uncomfortable and somebody asked if you had heard a joke, you may remember being reluctant to hear it at first. Before long you were probably totally absorbed in the joke, wondering what the punch line would be! Thirdly, the fact that humor can distract you is also very important because it helps you see things from a different perspective. Frequently, this can help you look at something more objectively, which may help you to handle it more effectively.

The ability to laugh at yourself is a very important part of maturing. How well this works, however, depends on what you are going through. It's nearly impossible (and probably ridiculous) to laugh at yourself when going through a crisis. Therefore, at the time of surgery, you would not be expected to laugh. However, as you adjust to having an ostomy, it becomes easier to laugh about it. Laugh at sounds (guess which ones!), laugh at experiences (don't guess which ones!), and that can help.

Relaxation Procedures

Relaxation is the opposite of tension. If you learn to relax, you will not be tense. But relaxation procedures, by themselves, will not control emotions. So why use them? Because if you feel more relaxed, you will be better able to identify those problems that are affecting you. You'll then be better able to figure out how to deal with them. So relaxation procedures can be the essential first steps in coping with your emotions.

How do you relax? This doesn't mean sitting in front of the television with a can of beer! There are different types of relaxation procedures. Progressive relaxation is a procedure in which you learn how to relax the muscles in your body. Hypnosis is another relaxation procedure, as is meditation and *the relaxation response*. There's also a procedure called *imagery*, where you select pictures in your mind that will help to relax you, thereby helping you to solve problems. More information about imagery can be found in the chapter, *Pain*. Books on any of these procedures are available in your local library, and can really help you to start feeling better.

Here's a quicky introduction to a relaxation procedure. I call it, appropriately, the quick release. First read the directions and then try it. Close your eyes, take a deep breath, and hold it while you tense or tighten every muscle in your body that you can think of (your fists, arms, legs, stomach, neck, buttocks, etc.). Hold your breath and muscle tension for about six seconds. Then let your breath out in a whoosh, and let your body go limp. Keep your eyes closed, and breathe rhythmically in and out for about 20 seconds. Repeat this tension/relaxation cycle three times. By the end of the third repetition, you'll probably feel a lot more relaxed.

Pinpointing

Now you're relaxed. So you're ready to proceed with the next crucial step. In order to deal effectively with anything that's upsetting you, you should determine exactly what's bothering you. Make a list. Then look over what you've written. Upon reviewing your list, you'll see that just about every item can be placed into one of two categories. The first category includes things (problems or emotions) you can do something about. The second category includes things you can't do anything about. Why separate them? Because the two categories have different implications for how to deal with them.

For the first category, things you can do something about, you'll want to figure out what strategies will help to improve the situation. You'll plan a course of action as soon as you identify exactly what's bothering you. How about the second category, things that you can't do anything about? You'll still be planning strategies, but of a different kind! Where does your feeling exist? In your mind, right? Therefore, for this category, you must work on the way you are thinking.

What Should You Do?

How can you change your thinking so that something will bother you less? Should you distract yourself? The technique you use really depends on what emotional reaction is bothering you. For example, if you're afraid of something, and you want to conquer this fear, a procedure called *systematic desensitization* may be helpful. You'll learn about this in the chapter, *Fears and Anxieties*.

If you feel guilty, angry, or depressed about something, it can be very helpful to learn how to change or "restructure" the way you're thinking. You'll learn more about such techniques in the chapters, *Guilt*, *Anger*, and *Depression*.

Actually, any of these procedures can be used with just about any problem. It's merely a question of deciding what approach is best for you in coping with your emotions.

WHAT ABOUT THE FUTURE?

Even if you have intense emotional reactions, they will soon diminish, either with time or because you're doing something to help. Of course, a range of emotional reactions may occur from time to time. Even if you had ostomy surgery years ago, you'll still feel a twinge of nostalgia, regret, or anxiety at times. But even when these feelings do occur, you can usually point to many things going on in your life that indicate your progress. This makes it easier to get past the unpleasantness. However, you won't be forever immune to negative feelings about ostomy surgery.

The purpose of this section is to help you to understand the different emotions you may experience, to learn where they come from, and, most importantly, to recognize that many ostomates have gone through exactly what you are now going through. In addition, different strategies will be presented to help you cope more effectively with these emotions.

In the following chapters, you'll see how these techniques can be used. So don't be afraid, depressed, guilty, or angry! Instead, read on!

7

Coping with the Diagnosis

When you first found out you needed ostomy surgery, how did you feel? How did you react when your doctor finally told you the news? You probably experienced one of two practically opposite types of reactions.

TYPE 1: WHAT A RELIEF!

One type of reaction is that of relief. Now, this may seem strange at first. Why would you be relieved to find out that you needed surgery? Well, maybe you were experiencing a lot of pain, and nothing seemed to help. Maybe your bowel habits had become so erratic that you had to schedule your whole life around them. Joanne, age 28, had gotten to the point where she could not go shopping in an unfamiliar store unless she knew there was a "multiple" stalled bathroom conveniently nearby. What a relief to know that surgery can remove this oppressive feeling! Maybe you went through a long period of time before being diagnosed. You might have gone from doctor to doctor, trying to find out once and for all what was really wrong with you, so you could begin treatment that would finally help you feel better. You may have been told by physicians or by friends and relatives that "it's all in your head." This can really be annoying! Maybe you were told that if you ate the proper foods and relaxed more the pain would go away. All you knew was that no "loving" remedies were helping the pain in your gut.

If you were relieved after being diagnosed, you probably had a much easier time coping with the surgery. Why? You may feel relief for several reasons. First, you're hopeful that ostomy surgery will drastically improve the way you've been feeling (and you finally know why you're feeling that way). Secondly, family members and friends who may not have believed that you were really sick can now learn the truth. Unfortunately, those close to you may still not believe that the problem is physical. They may still think that the problem is emotional or stress-related. You can't force everyone to believe in a medical diagnosis! However, most doubts will probably disappear (although they may be replaced by fear or uneasiness about your prognosis or about the ostomy itself). Relationships that may have been strained can improve. Sometimes, family members feel guilty, as they realize that they have been skeptical about your condition. They may have criticized your inability to fulfill responsibilities and your being less able to do things. They did this because they thought a real illness did not exist. Now they know! Thirdly, and most importantly, you'll be relieved that it wasn't all in your head. After a long time, even the most confident person can begin to wonder whether or not there is really something wrong or whether it is emotional.

TYPE 2: PANIC ATTACK!

The other, almost completely opposite, reaction is terror. Pure panic! You might have reacted, "Oh no, what are you going to do to me? Why do I need it? Will I ever be 'normal?' Will I ever get better? Am I going to die?" These are all tense questions that you may ask when you're diagnosed. Family members and loved ones may ask them, and panic, as well. You may feel that life will never be the same: it will now include an ostomy. This may further increase your panic.

Let's talk about this reaction. Who do you know who likes surgery? It's normal to be afraid. You may be hit with the fact that you are mortal, that you won't live forever. You may *not* be healthy for the rest of your life. Physically, it's not uncommon to feel faint, a shortness of breath, or to experience other stress reactions at the time of diagnosis.

WHY DID I FEEL CALM?

Frequently, as with any traumatic event, you may feel numb at first. You may sit quietly in the doctor's office, listening to everything that is said.

But you're not really absorbing it. You may hear your doctor talking, but it's not "sinking in." You might even actively and calmly participate in the discussion, without any emotional reaction. That may come later!

HOW ABOUT DENIAL?

Denying that a problem exists frequently occurs. Even if you've been experiencing prolonged and severe abdominal pain, being diagnosed as needing ostomy surgery may provoke denial. You may respond: "But I don't think I need surgery;" "I don't have this problem the way you think I do;" "Why don't you give it a little bit longer—I'm sure it will go away by itself;" or "★! (*) ×#, leave me alone!"

DEATH WISH (Charles Bronson, where are you?)

Did you ever wish you could die after being told you needed ostomy surgery? Some people do. They'd rather die than have part of their intestine removed. If you've ever felt this way, don't feel guilty. You're not alone. Furthermore, it will pass!

HOW DO YOU START TO ADJUST?

You must help yourself. Sure, you can get love and support from family and friends, and you can get expertise and support from professionals. But that's never enough. You are the one who must come to grips with having an ostomy. This is something you have to do yourself, regardless of what anyone else says or does. At first, adjusting may be a very difficult and ongoing struggle. It can require a lot of effort and understanding. You may go through a lot of emotional turmoil, but there is no other way. You must face it.

Information, please! Get as much as you can. Your physicians will be helpful in providing information, or at least suggesting ways for getting it. Next, read. Just make sure that your reading material is current. After reading general, consumer-oriented information, you may move to more technical material. Ask questions about anything you don't understand.

It probably wasn't your life-long goal to be an expert on your ostomy, but consider how this can help you. Doctors will respect your questions more. You'll understand exactly what's going on in your body. These are just two of the many advantages that come from reading about ostomies.

Should you believe everything you read? No. You may come across "cures" in weekly newspapers or magazines that sound incredible or alternatives to surgery that make you regret having had ostomy surgery. Make sure that whatever you read is reputable. Remember that it takes rigorous scientific study before a new procedure or even a treatment can be proven effective.

The best way to start coping with denial is by "reality testing." Speak to those professionals who know what your condition is and have them explain in further detail why these things are necessary. Look at any X-rays that have been taken. Talk to other people who have had the surgery and find out what they went through when first diagnosed. You will realize that many of their experiences parallel your own.

Supportive services and organizations have been established, specifically to provide you with all available information on ostomy surgery. Such organizations as the United Ostomy Association are invaluable in providing incredible amounts of information and support. They may also assist you in finding self-help groups, which can add to your knowledge of ostomy, as well as to your coping ability.

HOW ABOUT YOUR EMOTIONAL REACTION?

Try to consciously control any anxiety or stress that's making you uncomfortable. Once you realize that your body is now functioning differently, and altering your life-style, you'll want to try to control as many harmful emotions as you can.

It is very easy for your imagination to run wild. You'll probably think about everything that can go wrong. You'll worry about every symptom. If cancer were the reason for your surgery, you'd probably be frightened about how serious it can be, and how it can affect you and your family. Learn the facts about your condition. This is a great way to lessen some of the anxiety. Remember: everyone is different.

The emotions that arise from discovering the need for ostomy surgery can be upsetting. You may engage in prolonged periods of regret, sorrow, and nostalgia, remembering the way it used to be. Many fears come to mind, some of which can be overwhelming. Fear of incapacitation, of death, of being handicapped, of losing friends, are all very realistic. More about that in the chapter, *Fears and Anxieties*. Other chapters in this part of the book will help you to cope with other emotions, as well!

WHAT NEXT?

Once you've become more familiar with your ostomy and better understand how it affects you, what can you do to deal with it? Consult your E.T. Also, work with a physician you can trust, one who has had experience working with ostomates before, and can encourage you to feel that the patient-physician relationship you are developing will be very helpful later in life. Would you rather work with a physician who has had a lot of experience with ostomates, or with a very warm, friendly doctor, but one who is less familiar with ostomies? Most people prefer the former, but the choice is yours. Keep *your* goals in mind. Hopefully you can find a physician with both attributes!

Learn what specific changes may have to be made in your lifestyle. There is no way of knowing how many changes you'll have to make. Your goal is to create the best possible life for yourself.

Start facing your fears. They can and must be faced, in order to help your adjustment move along more smoothly. Speak to other people with ostomies. Learn how they've adjusted. This can be very helpful.

Did you ever ask yourself, "Why can't I go back to the way it used to be?" Have you wished you would wake up some morning and find out that this was all a bad dream? The more you keep hoping that all this will go away, the more you are slowing down your adjustment. Why does this slow it down? You're not really admitting to yourself that you've changed in a way that may last for the rest of your life. Rather, you're trying to push it out of your mind, hoping that things will return to the way they were. This makes it harder to cope with having an ostomy, since the problem is not being faced realistically. Try to accept the fact that your ostomy exists, that it is affecting you, and that it *will* remain with you. Try to plan all your activities and aim all your thinking towards the notion that you are going to do what you can to handle it effectively.

HOW ABOUT THE FAMILY?

A very important part of adjusting is having your family learn to adjust as well. It's so hard (for all) if family members around you have difficulty accepting your illness. Dealing with the diagnosis can be hard for family members. They also go through periods of denial, where they will say, "No, surgery is not necessary," or "I'm sure the problem will clear up by itself." Virginia, a 29-year-old secretary, had only recently been diagnosed as needing ostomy surgery. After a few depressing weeks, however, she had begun to cope. She was able to handle thoughts of body changes, alterations in bowel habits, and some of the other characteristics of having an ostomy. Great? No. Her husband of ten years wouldn't come near her, her children were afraid she was going to die, and even her 65-year-old mother was considering selling her condominium in Arizona to move closer. Although Virginia was learning how to cope with her ostomy, she was not able to cope with her family. *They* couldn't handle it.

It's a great idea for family members to look for people to speak to. They can find out more about ostomies and about how others cope with having a loved one with an ostomy. Family members can follow the suggestions given before: attending self-help groups, speaking to E.T.'s and physicians, and reading. Encourage family members and willing friends to learn about the ostomy. This will help you to adjust.

IN A NUTSHELL

Start thinking positively about moving on into the future. Learn as much as you can about your ostomy. Use whatever support systems are necessary to help you. Use all the stress management and emotional control procedures you can. Start saying to yourself, "I may have an ostomy, but I'm going to do whatever I can to help myself adjust to it." If it is necessary for you to make changes in your lifestyle, even major changes, tell yourself that you will do it, and do it willingly! You are going to lead as complete a life as you can. The more quickly you can adjust your lifestyle to fit your needs, the more rapidly you will be able to move on with the rest of your life. This may be hard. However, be grateful that you're not helpless!

8

Depression

George was depressed. A 41-year-old father of three, married for 18 years, he lived in a spacious home in an affluent neighborhood, and apparently had everything he could ask for—except an ostomy! He didn't ask for *that*. Whereas George had always been enthusiastic about life, he now found himself unhappy whenever he thought of the future. He felt that he could never again participate in sports and was afraid to see his friends. He didn't even want to spend time with his children. George was suffering from depression.

Depression is a serious problem. Mere mention of the word can sometimes wipe the smile right off your face. Actual numbers vary, but it is estimated that more than two million Americans need professional help for depression. Depression has been nicknamed the "common-cold" of emotional problems, since it is so widespread.

But what is depression? Depression is the extremely unpleasant feeling of unhappiness and despair. It can range from mild, where you may feel discouraged and downhearted, to severe, where you can feel utterly hopeless, worthless, and unwilling to go on with life. You may feel like there is no reason to remain a part of the world.

Depression can be painful. Imagine how it must hurt to feel (or say), "I wish I were never born. What good am I? I'm not helping anybody around me and I'm not helping myself." It may seem like life, and the whole world, are against you. Life is unfair, and a constant struggle in which there is never a victory. That hurts.

DEPRESSION AFFECTS YOUR BODY

The most noticeable symptoms of depression may be physical. Nervous activity or agitation, such as wringing the hands, may occur. You may be restless, or have difficulty remaining in one place. On the other hand, you may become much less active, and remain motionless for abnormally long periods of time (appearing almost catatonic, with no apparent desire to do anything). Not wanting to do anything is common in depression. Patty became very concerned when her 32-year-old husband, Jack, remained sitting in the living room for hours at a time. When she asked him a question, he would respond in monosyllables. When people phoned to talk to him, he never took the calls. Jack's depression was causing him to lose interest in just about everything.

Other physical changes that can occur are a reduction (or sometimes an increase) in appetite, a decreased interest in sex, and, for some women, a ceasing of menstruation. If you're mildly depressed, you may have difficulty concentrating, and have a much shorter attention span. When you speak (you'll probably do less of that, too) your conversation may be shallow, often emphasizing feelings of worthlessness and hopelessness. Most of your physical activities will slow down.

You'll probably feel exhausted. This may be surprising, since you're hardly doing anything. But constantly telling yourself that you're no good can even be tiring! You really don't want to believe this, but you feel you have no choice. In trying to escape from these feelings, you may become even more depressed, as well as more physically drained and exhausted.

Feeling depressed may make you feel sick physically as well. This is due to the many ways your body reacts when you are depressed. Any one of the symptoms we've talked about could be indicative of a physical disorder. The symptoms may go away when your depression improves. However, don't just accept the fact that they are related to depression. A medical examination may still be a good idea. This way, you'll make sure that there is no organic disease causing your depression.

DEPRESSION AFFECTS YOUR MOOD

You may experience mood swings. Sometimes, you'll feel worse in the morning and better in the evening. This isn't unusual, since evening means it is almost time to go to sleep, the great "escape." On the other hand, you may have some difficulty sleeping, making night a dreaded part of the day.

When you feel depressed, your mood keeps getting "lower." You like yourself very little, if at all. Your thinking is very negative, very different from the way it is when you're feeling okay. It is such negative thinking, not just a particular triggering event, which leads to your depression. This negative thinking tends to be the most frequently overlooked or misunderstood part of depression. Recognizing this is an important first step in learning to cope with depression.

DEPRESSION AFFECTS RELATIONSHIPS

When you're depressed, you may feel that people around you have no need for you. As George used to complain, "Why should my friends want to see me or make plans with me?"

Do you feel less at ease talking to others? Do others seem to be having difficulty talking to you, even if they have been close to you for a long time? You may feel less interested in conversation, and less confident. You may project *your* own feelings of self-worthlessness onto others, believing that they really don't want to talk to you. The more depressed you are, the more persuasive you may be in convincing others that you are no good.

Heather received a telephone call from her friend, who wanted to know how she had been feeling, since she hadn't seen her at work for several days. Heather responded very half-heartedly, "knowing" that her friend was calling out of obligation. She then explained that she would understand if her friend did not want to call, because she never had any good news to tell her. She knew that if she were in the same position, she wouldn't want to hear such bad news all the time. Therefore, she would not hold it against her friend if she no longer called. How do you think her friend felt? Imagine hearing this repeatedly, despite reassuring Heather that her concern was sincere. Eventually, *anyone* would get tired of even trying, and would probably stop calling. What would this do? In Heather's mind, it would reinforce the fact that she really was no good, and was not worthy of having friends.

DEPRESSION AFFECTS PHYSICAL ACTIVITIES

Do you find that you are getting less satisfaction from your normal activities? Are you functioning like an automaton? Does something seem to be missing? It can be depressing to realize that something you used to enjoy is no longer giving you the same pleasure, especially if you don't know why. It almost seems like you are being forced to go through the motions. Your heart just isn't in it. It is understandable, therefore, that if you are depressed, you might prefer not doing anything. This is better than participating in something from which you would derive no pleasure.

What happens after that first depressing event occurs? A kind of chain reaction follows. This one event creates a feeling that spreads like wildfire. It's almost as if the "bottom drops out." You may feel less in control of your thinking (this is not true, as we will see later), and that you are "destined" to end in the deepest pit. But keep in mind that, the deeper you go into depression, the harder it is to climb back up again. Therefore, it is certainly desirable to identify these feelings of depression as early as possible, to try and keep yourself from spiraling further downward.

WHAT CAUSES DEPRESSION?

Where does depression come from? Sometimes we can figure it out, sometimes we can't. But before we give up, let's discuss some of the possible causes!

How About the Normal "Downs"?

A certain amount of depression is normal in anyone's life. Nobody's life is constantly an "upper." We all experience normal cycles of ups and downs. If we didn't experience some of the downs, we could never fully appreciate the ups! It is when depression becomes more than the normal "downs" that it must be attended to. Nipping it quickly can keep it from becoming a much deeper depression.

Certain things in anyone's life can understandably lead to depression. Certain traumatic experiences, such as losing a loved one, being diagnosed with a chronic illness, requiring major surgery, being fired from a job—all may certainly lead to depression. That would be understandable. However, this *doesn't* mean you should ignore it or wait until it goes away. It's essential to learn how to deal with depression, since this is so important in learning how to cope with an ostomy.

How About Anger You Can't Express?

What if you get so angry that you feel like you're going to burst? Because you don't (or can't) do anything about it, you "swallow" it. It seems strange that a powerful feeling like anger can become a withdrawn, helpless feeling like depression. But it does. You can get depressed if you bottle anger inside you. If you become increasingly angry about something, and feel unable to do anything about it, you may turn the anger inward. You may feel so much frustration or hopelessness that you "shut down" in an attempt to keep yourself from these terrible feelings. This leads you to withdraw.

Is it All in Our Heads?

A small percentage of depression cases may be caused by a biochemical deficiency or some chemical imbalance in the body. This does not occur very often. Treatment for a biochemical deficiency may involve the administration of drugs in an effort to re-balance body chemicals. This is usually only part of the answer. Yet, regardless of whether or not your depression is caused by this (or by the more common reactions to things, people, and events around you), you should still try to modify your behavior and improve your thinking. Experts believe that, even if the cause of depression *is* biochemical, improving your thoughts and behavior can have a positive effect on you.

How About Ostomy?

How can having an ostomy cause depression? Are you kidding? Having an ostomy can certainly create, or magnify, depression.

Any depression you might have felt at the time of surgery is understandable. It usually lessens as you become more adjusted to your new life situation. The fact that it takes a long time to adjust to having the ostomy, however, is a problem when you consider what depression can do to you. So if your depression lingers, don't wait until you've fully adjusted to the "new you" before learning how to cope with it.

You may be saying to yourself, "If I'm depressed because I have an ostomy, how can I expect to get over my depression unless I no longer have an ostomy?" That kind of thinking will get you nowhere. We'll talk more later about how you can improve your thinking.

What else might depress you about having an ostomy? You might get depressed about the future, now knowing what your prognosis is, or how it will affect your life. The way your body feels or looks may depress you. Necessary changes in habits created by the ostomy may also be depressing.

Other people may upset and depress you. You may feel helpless at not being able to really talk about what you're experiencing or how you feel. You may get depressed over others' lack of understanding or sympathy (of course, you don't want to be pitied, either!). You may be depressed over the possibility of damaged relationships, lost friendships, or family friction. If you're single, you may become depressed by thinking that you'll never meet anyone, or develop a meaningful relationship.

WHAT MAINTAINS DEPRESSION?

Why do you stay depressed? Why doesn't it just go away? It may be because you don't want to talk to anybody, or to even consider getting some therapy. Therefore, the feelings that have led to your depression tend to be kept hidden. How, then, can anything be done about them? It would probably be helpful (even though you wouldn't be too thrilled) if somebody around you took the initiative and forced you into some kind of conversation (therapeutic or otherwise) or, at least, into physical activities.

You may ask, "Is my unwillingness to talk the only reason why I'm still depressed? If I start talking more, will that get me out of my depression?" Not necessarily. You may be blaming yourself (or the ostomy) for everything that is wrong. You may become more and more withdrawn, pulling away from the world around you. Why? Well, if you feel your ostomy is doing all of these horrible things, isn't it better to "escape," to not think about it? Objectively, escaping doesn't solve anything. But if you're depressed, you may feel that the only way to solve this dilemma is by withdrawing. This keeps you depressed—in fact, it can make you even more depressed.

To others you may seem apathetic and withdrawn, but I know you're in deep, emotional pain. I'm not talking about any physical discomfort from your ostomy. It also hurts to feel depressed or worthless. Part of what makes you, and keeps you, depressed is your effort to protect yourself from this emotional pain. When your mind does allow any thoughts to enter, these tend to be feelings of doom and destruction, feelings that nothing good can possibly happen, that only bad things can happen. So, what do you do? You try to block everything out of your mind!

HOW DO WE DEAL WITH DEPRESSION?

Can anything be done? Of course! Would I abandon you in such a time of despair? First, tell yourself that the *main* reason you're still depressed is because you have not yet taken those beneficial steps that can help you to feel better! These steps can "bring you out of your rut" and reacquaint you with the more positive, pleasant apsects of living. Don't think it's easy, though. Unfortunately, once you have become depressed, it takes effort, hard work, and a certain amount of persistance to pull yourself back up. The fight, however, is surely worth it. Of course, the fight can be made easier, knowing specific techniques and activities that will help. I'm sure you realize that, once you feel better, you're not going to ever want to feel so depressed again. Take heart in knowing that the most effective strategies and techniques in dealing with depression can also help prevent you from becoming depressed again. This doesn't mean you'll never feel depressed again. But if it does happen, isn't it nice to know that you can fight it? You *can* do something to help yourself.

TYPES OF DEPRESSION TREATMENT

Now that you're ready to fight your depression, consider two major ways of dealing with it: being more physical (in other words, *doing* something), and working on your thinking.

It can be very helpful to make a list of everything that depresses you. You may feel there will be at least 50 items, right? In actuality, you'll probably start running dry after six or seven. Divide this list into two more lists: things that you *can do* something about, and things you *can't* do anything about. Get physical (do something) about those items on the first list, and get thoughtful (work on your thinking) concerning items on the second list.

Let's Get Physical

You may be using a lot of energy to keep yourself depressed. You may be working hard to keep that anger inside, even if it seems like you are withdrawing. If depression is often inwardly - turned anger, then releasing this anger can eliminate feelings of depression. But what do you do with those feelings of anger? You must find an object to express your anger towards. This may be difficult if there is another person who you are really angry at. You may be unable to express your feelings in a way that will release your anger, or do anything constructive to help you feel better. However, it is important to release the trapped anger in an effort to keep it from building up and deepening the depression.

Have you ever experienced the following? You're sitting there, depressed and withdrawn. Somebody makes an innocent remark, and you practically snap the person's head off! What's happening is that whatever was said triggered the release of some of the internalized anger that was making you depressed. Look out, world!

It takes an awful lot of energy to keep you depressed. Learn to release this energy outwardly. What kinds of activities can be helpful for this? Jogging or other intense physical activity can be good. Bicycle riding, running, or playing tennis are all activities that require a great expenditure of energy and can result in some lifting of depression. Physical activity is not the only way to ease depression, however. Thank goodness, right? But there are other reasons why, even if you like to participate in physical activities, this may not be the best way for you to eliminate depression. What if you're so depressed that you don't *feel* like being physical? Who's going to make you? Nobody will force you, you won't force yourself, and you'll just continue to lie there in a depressed heap. Another reason is that, although getting physical may lessen your depression, it's your *feelings* that make you depressed. Physical activity can be a great distraction, and can help you to look more objectively at what's going on. That will help. But it may not teach you what you need the most: ways of fighting inappropriate thinking. "Getting physical" may not help you to control subsequent feelings that can make you depressed all over again.

Let's Get Thoughtful

By now you've realized that, just as you may "think" yourself into depression, you can "think" yourself out of depression. How? Your thoughts show how you "talk to yourself." You're always telling yourself things. In fact, when it comes to talking to yourself, you're probably the biggest chatterbox you know! But if you're depressed, you're just talking yourself down. All your thoughts (or at least most of them) are put-downs, or harsh statements giving you little to be happy about. This doesn't help you to feel better; instead, it can make you even more depressed. You want your inner chatterbox to help you, not hurt you. Let's see how you can do that.

Separating Fact from Fiction

Don't get defensive when I say: if you are depressed, you probably tend to distort reality. Clinical research with depressed patients has proven this. Recognize, therefore, that what you are thinking is not necessarily based on what is really going on, but on your own distorted views. What you're doing is called *cognitive distortion*. Uh oh! Is that bad? You bet your happiness it is.

Cognitive refers to your thinking. *Distortion* means you're twisting things around, and losing sight of what's real. We all do this from time to time. But when you're depressed, you do it *a lot*, if not all the time, and it *keeps* you depressed. So, how do you stop? First, you must become reacquainted with what is really happening. But how can you do that if you are distorting reality? Right now, you're better off accepting somebody *else's* perceptions of what's going on, because that person is probably a lot more accurate. Since so many of the feelings of worthlessness that characterize depression are based on distorted facts, depression can be reduced, even eliminated, if these facts are straightened out.

Margie was depressed because none of her friends ever called. "They don't call as much as they used to before I had my surgery. They don't care. That depresses me," she would whine. Her sister, Melissa, asked her to estimate how often her friends called before surgery. When she compared this to the number of calls she was receiving now, Margie realized that the numbers were nearly the same. She then realized she was probably just more sensitive to this! Although she did not feel completely better, she did feel better knowing that she wasn't being abandoned.

Making Molehills out of Mountains

Does this imply that if you're depressed you have no real problems? Is it "all in your head?" No. Every person has problems, both big and small. If you are feeling o.k., you can handle these problems. If you're feeling depressed, you may feel overwhelmed. Each and every part of your life, regardless of how trivial or slight, tends to depress you. As the depression lifts, you will again be able to deal with *all* of life's problems.

Self-Fulfilling Prophecy

We've discussed several different feelings that you may have if you are depressed. Are all of these feelings irrational and untrue? No. Ironically, although some of them may start off being far from the truth, the longer you feel that way the greater chance they have of becoming "self-fulfilling prophecies." In other words, you'll convince yourself that such nonsense makes sense. For example, if you start telling yourself that friends and relatives don't care, this may become a reality because your depression and negative attitudes may alienate the people close to you. It may be so much harder for them to be with you that they may feel, "why bother?" As far as your activities go, because you are depressed you are less likely to do anything. You probably won't even attempt doing things that you may have wanted to do once. As a result, you'll feel less competent. You'll know you are not accomplishing anything. This just magnifies and confirms your feelings of worthlessness, which leads to even more depression. Not a pretty picture.

Once you begin feeling depressed, your negative thoughts will lead to more negative actions, and so on. This will just spiral you downward into more and more extreme depression. Eventually, you will feel trapped, that there is no way for you to escape from the "dumps." You'll find yourself engulfed in this vicious cycle.

Are you getting depressed just reading this? If you have been, or are depressed, you've probably said to yourself at least once already, "Wow, that sounds just like me!" So you see, you're not alone. What can be done? The rule is: *don't* let your negative thoughts become self-fulfilling prophecies. If you become aware that you are starting to believe in negative thoughts, stop yourself. Try to set up positive thoughts in your mind, so that if your thought does turn out to be real, it will be the positive one, instead.

Positive is the Opposite of Negative

As mentioned previously, depression results from, and causes, a lot of negative thinking. Negative thoughts automatically pop into your head and can't be stopped. It's like trying to keep your eyes open when you sneeze! But once you become aware of them, you *can* do something. People who remain depressed feel incapable of doing anything and allow negative thoughts to continue. They continue in this vicious, downward cycle, which leads to more severe depression. But when you feel o.k., on the other hand, you are able to counteract these negative automatic thoughts.

Ann, a 34-year-old housewife, was resting one day when the telephone rang. "I'm sure that's Katherine, calling to cancel our lunch plans," was the thought that immediately popped into her mind. Within the 30 seconds it took her to get to the phone, she had become so depressed that she considered not even answering it so she wouldn't hear the bad news. Imagine how she felt when she reluctantly answered the phone, only to find out it was the wrong number! Ann had allowed her negative thoughts to run wild—she became more and more negative until she was ready to give up. And for what? There was no clear-cut reason for continuing her negative thought.

Once she realized she was thinking this way, what should she have done? She should have *reversed* her thoughts. She should have told herself, "It may not even be Katherine on the phone. Or, if it is, maybe she's just calling to confirm. I won't let it get to me now. I don't even know who it is." This is a step toward turning negative thoughts into positive ones.

Dwell on the Brighter Tomorrows

If you find yourself unhappily comparing your present life to life before surgery, try to modify your thinking by planning fun things for the present and future. Anyone can come up with some enjoyable things to do, regardless of how restricted you may be. But it takes effort. Don't wallow in self-pity, because that allows your depression to strangle you. Work on your thinking, develop some positive plans, and translate that into fun, pleasure, and saying goodby to your depression.

When you think about the past, you may not always think about how much better it was. You may have been in constant pain. Or you may have had to severely restrict your schedule because of intestinal problems. You may be upset about mistakes you've made, ways in which you "fell down in life." But these thoughts may make you feel hopeless about the future. How depressing! However, you can't change the past. What's done is done. Tell yourself that—repeatedly. Tell yourself that you're going to work on making the future more successful. Think about specific goals. Start with those that are easy-to-reach. You'll feel like you're helping yourself just by thinking about what you can do to help. Don't punish yourself for the past.

What's Missing in your Life?

You may have laughed when you read this subtitle. "Health," you might say. "Part of my intestinal or urinary tract." Sure. But why discuss this? Because depressed people frequently lament the fact that something is missing from their lives. Usually what is missing is a feeling of satisfaction, and the feeling of praise and warmth that you get from other people. You may just miss people being nice to you, being interested in you, paying attention to you. This may make you feel worthless. How do you counteract this? Think about your positive qualities (you do have some!) Think about how you can interact more with people, spark their interest, and get more of that satisfaction that makes you feel so worthwhile.

Shoot for the Earth, Not the Moon

We all have goals. It's only natural to get upset when we don't reach a particular one, especially if we've tried very hard to get there. But maybe it's not a goal that is realistically within reach. Maybe you're trying to do something you can't, and you're getting depressed instead of realistically resetting your goal.

Regina had not returned to work since her surgery six weeks previously. She made it through her recuperation period, knowing she'd feel better when she got back to work and caught up on everything she had to do. When her doctor finally gave her the go-ahead, she practically flew there. After two hours of phone calls, typing, dictation, and meetings, she was exhausted. Her feelings plummeted. She didn't think she could make it. She felt that her surgery would cost her her job. She had simply set her sights too high. Expecting to do everything as if you had never been sick is just not realistic. It's better to try a more gradual return to work. Slide into your old activities slowly. Build up your stamina. The end result is more important, isn't it? And if your goals are more realistically set, you've got a much better chance of achieving them, and a smaller chance of being depressed about falling short.

AN ANTI-DEPRESSING SUMMARY

So the best way to work on negative thoughts is to prevent them from continuing, not from occurring. Be more positive and realistic. Deal with reality the way it truly exists. Deal with thoughts from a more factual point of view. Think about the way somebody else may see them, somebody who can be more objective, and who isn't depressed. Try to make your perceptions more accurate, your awareness more realistic, and your thoughts more positive and constructive. Remember: your thoughts lead to your emotions. If your thoughts are negative and critical, your emotions will be in bad shape. However, if you can turn your thoughts around to a more positive, constructive point of view, then your emotional reactions will improve as well.

9

Fears and Anxieties

Don't be "afraid" to read this chapter! It may help you learn what you're "anxious" about!

Those two sentences may help you to distinguish between fear and anxiety. What's the difference? *Anxiety* is a general sense of uneasiness, a vague feeling of discomfort. It is an agitated, uncertain state where you just don't feel at peace or in control. There is a premonition that something bad may happen, which you have to protect yourself against. You feel very vulnerable. You're not sure exactly what the source of your anxiety is.

Fear, on the other hand, is usually more specific. It's often directed towards something that we can recognize, be it a person, an object, a situation, or an event. We have fear when we become aware of something dangerous, or when we feel threatened. When we are afraid, as with feeling anxious, we also feel like we are not in control. We feel less confident in ourselves. So the *feelings* of fear and anxiety are basically the same. The difference, for the most part, is whether or not you can identify the source of the feeling. From this point on, though, let's use the two terms interchangeably.

Fear is so prevalent that many different words are used to describe it: scared, concerned, worried, uptight, nervous, edgy. Then there's perplexity, having cold feet, feeling insecure, helpless, frustrated. Is that it? Nope! How about suspicious, keyed-up, impatient, giddy, hesitant, apprehensive, tense, disturbed, agitated. Of course, there are more, but if I went on this book would have to be renamed, "The Fear Synonym Book." All these words mean the same thing: "I'm afraid." The source of this fear may be real or imaginary.

IS FEAR GOOD OR BAD?

Believe it or not, fear is usually good! Now you're probably saying, "If I'm shaking with fear, how can it be good?" Fear mobilizes you. It "tells" you to prepare to attack the source of your fear. You react in a way that leads to action. In this regard, fear is similar to stress. It serves a necessary and critical purpose. In a way, it "protects" you.

Fear is bad only if it is denied, or if it is so excessive that you can't do anything about it. If you face it and push past it, trying to resolve it, then fear is a positive emotion. It is only when the source of fear becomes overlooked, ignored, or denied that the consequences may be a problem. This is because the threat or danger is allowed to continue, and nothing (or not enough) is being done to control it.

HOW INTENSE ARE OUR REACTIONS?

Fear ranges in intensity from mild to severe. It is impossible to measure how much fear there is in anyone's life. It is unique and varies from person to person.

What determines how fearful you get? Usually, the strength of the feared object, person, or event is important. Also, how close is it (wouldn't you be more afraid of getting an injection within the next 30 seconds, than if you were getting it in 30 days)? How vulnerable are you (do you *hate* injections, or are you just tired of feeling like a pin-cushion)? How successful are you in defending yourself (can you calmly accept the needle, or do you scream a lot)? These are some of the factors determining how you handle fear. Your own strength and the success of your defense mechanisms also play a role.

Bobbi, age 28, was afraid to go to sleep at night. She was worried that she'd wake up in the morning with a recurrence of her embarrassing leakage problem. She felt fine at night, knowing she had made it through another day with no leakage. Therefore, she didn't want to go to sleep. What if Bobbi were stronger emotionally? She might still be concerned about this happening, but would not let it disturb her sleep. However, Bobbi *wasn't* strong. She was frightened. This fear kept her awake. Her restlessness might have even increased the possibility of the very problem she wanted to avoid!

People with ostomies can be afraid of many things. Obviously, the more fears you have, the more these can interfere with your successful adjustment. Recognizing your fears and learning how to deal with them will help you live more happily and more comfortably. How? I thought you'd never ask!

HOW TO COPE WITH FEARS AND ANXIETIES

The first step in coping with your fears is to use the "pinpointing" technique discussed in Chapter 6. List all the things you're afraid of. Identify exactly what you are afraid of and exactly why you are afraid. Then think about what you can do to alleviate your fears.

For Janine, this was not hard. She knew she was afraid of what people would say when they heard she had surgery. She realized that what she feared most was rejection. Perhaps people wouldn't want to be with her because of their own fears ("Could this happen to me?"). She planned a course of action (no, not a one-way ticket to Brazil). She decided to walk with her head held high, and *expect* her friends to accept her the way she was. If they didn't, that was *their* loss. She was less afraid almost instantly. As you begin planning your strategies, and gradually put your plan into operation, you'll continue to feel better and better.

Desensitize Yourself

A great technique used to conquer fears is called *systematic desensitization.* You learn to desensitize yourself to make yourself less vulnerable to the source of your fear.

Sit in a comfortable chair and relax. Then create a movie in your mind. Imagine what it is that makes you afraid. If you get tense, stop imagining it and relax. Then try imagining it again. The more you try to imagine your fear, the less it will bother you. Try it! It will give you a great feeling of relaxation and control. There are library books that give more information on systematic desensitization. Check them out.

It was stated earlier that anxiety is a vague, uneasy feeling with an unknown source. So how can you cope with it by following the steps listed above? Well, if you try to pinpoint the source and are unable to, then you can't follow the steps. So what do you do? Use relaxation procedures. Work on changing your thinking. Even if you can't pinpoint a specific fear, these techniques will greatly help you to cope with anxiety.

LET'S TALK ABOUT SPECIFICS

Remember, it is understandable for you to have many fears before surgery, after surgery, and even when you're back in good physical shape. A problem, however, arises when you don't admit these fears. As a result, you don't do anything about resolving them. They *can* be resolved. And you *can* work on changing your thinking.

Initial Fears

When you were first diagnosed, many fearful questions probably came to mind. "What will the future be like? What will become of me? What will people think? Will I die?" These are all legitimate questions and justifiable fears. But time goes on. Some of these questions have been answered, and some of your initial qualms have not materialized. But you're probably still afraid of some things. Let's discuss some of them.

Fear of Dying

This can occur any time someone goes through major surgery. Fear of dying is understandable. Or perhaps you have felt you were going to die of pain, anguish, or even embarrassment! Surgery was performed to help you live longer, not to make you die sooner. Improved surgical techniques and medical knowledge have significantly lowered the mortality rate. That may be reassuring, but it doesn't mean that this common fear won't cross your mind.

When might you be most afraid of dying? Probably at the time of diagnosis. That's when you feel the most vulnerable. Or perhaps at a time when your symptoms are particularly rough. Post-surgical treatment, reminding you of your vulnerability, can also cause these fears. When you *feel* the worst, you're most likely to *fear* the worst. However, being afraid of dying is not going to help you feel better or live longer. If anything, it's only going to make you feel worse! Being afraid of dying, therefore, falls into the category of fears that you can do little or nothing about. Think positively. Others have had worse symptoms and still live comfortably. Do you see how you must work on your thinking? If negative thoughts make you *more* afraid, then positive thoughts . . . !

When you're feeling better, and have fewer symptoms, you're less likely to be as afraid of dying. At that point, however, you're more likely to be afraid of other things.

Fear of Cancer

Fear of cancer is very common in many people, and is further intensified if cancer was the cause of your surgery in the first place. Most people can push cancer thoughts away. But if you were diagnosed as needing ostomy surgery because of cancer, you'll certainly have this fear. Remind yourself once again that surgery was designed to help your condition. With proper post-surgical treatment, your chances for licking the disease are improved. If your fears continue, be sure to get some professional help.

Fear of Pain

Nobody likes pain. Ostomy surgery should help to reduce chronic intestinal pain, but post-surgical discomfort is common. You may be afraid of the pain. This fear may be just as strong when you *don't* have pain, since you're afraid of it happening! If you do feel pain, you'll wonder when you're going to feel some relief. Each little twinge of pain may make you fear the need for more surgery or that other problems still exist. What can you do about this fear? Try to accept the fact that some pain may be "with you" from time to time, but medication can reduce its intensity. Realize that the pain will eventually stop or at least ease up. It *won't* last forever.

Fear of "What Next?"

What will happen next? You can't be sure. Will there be a recurrence of
the problem causing surgery? Will there be a problem with the stoma?
Fear of "what next?" includes being afraid of new symptoms, or the return
of old ones. Everyone *wonders* what's in store for the future. But because of
the unpleasantness of what you've experienced, you may be *afraid* of the
future, rather than merely curious. What can you do? Unless you own a
crystal ball, you can't foresee what will happen in the future. So take life
one day at a time. What will be, will be. (What a great name for a song!)
Any problems will be handled as they occur.

Fear of the View

Some ostomates are afraid to even look at their stomas or, perish the
thought, their stomas in action. Just thinking about this may cause you to
grimace. In the past, how many of you looked lovingly into the bowl before flushing? There is no real need for you to spend time looking at the
waste matter you've excreted. But you'll certainly be more aware of it. If
this bothers you, try using desensitization procedures to gradually get used
to this.

Ostomy surgery has created a whole new maintenance problem. Now,
in addition to brushing your teeth and combing your hair, you must be
more intimately involved in the elimination of body wastes than ever before. You may fear touching excrement or urine. You may fear the
lengthy amount of time necessary for elimination. So what should you
do? Remind yourself that, as with anything new, it takes time to get used
to it.

Give yourself a chance. Discuss your fears with professionals or other
ostomates. You'll feel better just knowing you're not the only one who has
felt this way.

Fear of Disability

The thought of being disabled may be horrible. Having an ostomy
shouldn't be disabling (after recovery). But that doesn't mean you won't

be afraid of this. Being "disabled" is a bad term, since it suggests that you can't do *anything*. If you look around you or think more objectively, you'll realize that a physical disability wouldn't make you any less of a human being. You would still have many, many capabilities. Numerous Olympic champions began their athletic careers to overcome physical disabilities. Beethoven wrote some of his greatest music after becoming totally deaf. There was even a one-armed baseball player in the major leagues. Regardless of their disabilities, these people have one thing in common: the knowledge that they can overcome or at least compensate for a limitation in one area by developing abilities in another. So, although it is unlikely that your ostomy will drastically curtail your physical activities, you can use these more positive thoughts to help you cope with this fear.

Fear of Appliance Malfunction

Are you afraid of leakage? Are you afraid that your appliance will not work the way it's supposed to? The more of an expert you become in caring for your appliance, the less fear you'll have. Initially, you may want to carry extra supplies with you, just in case. The best way to alleviate this fear is to become skilled in methods of attaching appliances, changing them, and maintaining them. You can always practice! The more experience you have, the more confidence you will gain as well.

Fear of Others' Reactions

Are you afraid that other people will not accept you with an ostomy (if they know about it)? Do you fear being shunned? Accept the fact that some people can be cold and unfeeling and may have trouble dealing with the "new" you. Who needs those kinds of friends, anyway? Other friends will accept you under any circumstances. Enjoy them. But since you can't change the way others feel, try not to be as concerned with reactions. Instead, be more attentive to your own needs and feelings.

Other fears in this category can be even more frightening. "What if my spouse leaves me? . . . What if friends stay away from me?" Isolation can be a horrible thought. If it's not happening now, you may be afraid of it happening in the future. You may be afraid that none of your friends will remain "in your corner." To reduce the chances of such rejection, you may hesitate to make plans with friends or family. This would only add to your feeling of isolation.

Consider your thoughts, but consider them realistically. Then realize that a change in a social relationship can occur for *any* reason, not just because of your ostomy! If you feel that your relationship is in jeopardy, see what you can do to help ("put all your cards on the table," discuss problems, even get counseling, if need be). You can only do so much. If that doesn't work, even though the outcome may upset you, at least you know you've tried.

Fear of Overdoing / Underdoing

You may not know how much you should do. You may be afraid of doing too much, but you may feel guilty about doing too little! How do you conquer this? Get advice from your doctor, or E.T. Don't overdo, especially right after surgery. Eventually, learning how much you should do will become largely a matter of trial-and-error. You can only learn through experience. Pace yourself. Change your level of activity gradually. Then tell yourself, as with so many other fears, that you're doing the best you can.

Fear of Going Out

Are you afraid to go out? You may think you're going to have an accident or that some sounds or odors may attract undesired attention. Maybe you're afraid that you won't find restroom facilities when you need them. Maybe you're concerned about how others will look at you or treat you. It is understandable to be afraid of these things, but does that mean you should stay home all the time? That won't help you to overcome these fears. You *can* do something to help them—plan ahead! Use the systematic desensitization techniques that we discussed earlier. Imagine all those terrible things happening, repeatedly, and their fear-value will diminish. Amusingly ask yourself, "What's the worst that could happen?" Then imagine your appliance exploding while you're shopping, and other shoppers racing out of the store, trampling each other in an attempt to outrun the waves of feces flowing through the store aisles! Or imagine a leakage problem causing a disgusting odor. Picture everyone near you starting to point at you, grimacing and holding their noses. Yes, these thoughts are unpleasant, but they probably made you smile. If you imagine them vividly enough, you'll be able to put things into better perspective. You'll see that these situations need not be so threatening.

Fear of Working

You may be concerned about whether or not you'll be able to keep your job. You may want to work, but fear that you won't be able to. Your employer may be understanding at first, but you worry about how long this will continue. Can you do much to change the nature of fear? Nope. You may even be afraid to tell your employer about your ostomy. Why should you? You may feel that you have a better chance of keeping your job by not saying anything. If it is not already known, your employer will probably never realize it anyway.

Fear of Clothing

No, this doesn't mean that you've become deathly afraid of touching or seeing clothing. Nor does it mean that you'll be nervous unless you go around naked! Rather, you may never want to appear in public again because you're afraid you'll have to wear bulky clothes to protect yourself. You may also fear the protrusion of appliances through clothing, and believe that other people will be able to look at you and instantly know why you look the way you do!

At the age of 28, Sue Anne had ileostomy surgery to treat her Crohn's disease. She immediately expressed the fear that she'd never again be able to wear the beautiful clothes she loved. "I don't want to look like I'm wearing rags," she would moan. But she felt she had no choice. If you have had this fear, here's a great solution. Go to a meeting of ostomates, and look at the styles being worn. You'll see people as well-dressed and as stylish as those at any other meeting you might attend. You'll probably even have difficulty distinguishing between the ostomate and the family member! This can certainly open up your eyes (to say nothing about your clothing budget!) You'll see that your clothes can be "chic" after all. You'll just have to wait until your recovery is complete.

Fear of Traveling

You may be reluctant to travel with an ostomy. Why? What if you have a problem while you're away, and you're not properly equipped? Obviously, traveling by car isn't so bad. You'll be able to bring extra supplies, and you're not going to be so far away that you couldn't get help if you really needed it. But you might be afraid to fly somewhere for a vacation. You wouldn't know the doctors, what medical facilities were available, or who you could contact if you experienced a problem.

What can you do? By planning in advance, you should be able to conquer this fear. Ask your doctor if he knows of any doctors or facilities where you're planning to go. You might want to contact them in advance. If your physician has no contacts, try to get some names either on your own (try the local medical society, or your local Ostomy Association), or plan your vacation at a place where adequate medical services are available. Take extras of every type of supply you use, and plan on not overdoing. Visiting five landmarks in one day is a bit much! More about this in the chapter, *Traveling*.

Fear of Not Coping

You may feel that you're barely handling having an ostomy. You may think that any new problem that comes along will be enough to push you over the edge. Fear of falling apart can easily lead to panic; an out-of-control kind of feeling that *will* make you fall apart. Get a hold of yourself. Pinpoint those particular things you're having difficulty with, and get help in dealing with them. Don't wait. Don't project a false sense of bravado that you can and must handle everything yourself. If you feel yourself near the edge, get someone to help you to steady yourself. Talk it over with someone. Once you share your feelings and fears with someone, you may see things a little more clearly. You may be able to deal with problems with greater strength, knowing that you're not alone. Once you're back in control, this fear will disappear.

A FEARLESS SUMMARY

Although many different fears have been discussed in this chapter, we have probably not covered all of the ones you have experienced. In addition, the coping suggestions offered certainly do not include all possible ways of dealing with fear. So what should you do?

You're working on recognizing your fears, right? For some of them, you're modifying your behavior. For others, you're modifying your thinking. Soon you will feel more in control. As this happens, you'll notice your fears begin to diminish. That doesn't mean that they'll all go away. But as you work on them and feel more in control, they'll at least lessen in intensity. You'll feel better knowing that you can do something about some of them, and that you're capable of handling them.

10

Anger

For years, 26-year-old Louise had been dying for an invitation to the neighborhood "splash" party, the "in" event of the year. Only a special group was invited. This year, Louise had finally received her gilt-edged invitation. How did she react? By tearing it into a thousand pieces and throwing it away, screaming and crying the whole time. Why? Louise recently had ileostomy surgery for Crohn's disease, and there was no way she wanted to show up at a swim party. Louise was angry!

This may have been the wrong reaction, however. Louise was not obligated to swim, or even to "suit up" at this party. In addition, she should have realized that many fashionable one-piece bathing suits give no indication of the wearer's condition. Instead of getting so angry, Louise should have considered alternatives. Get some tape for that invitation, Louise!

Regardless of the outcome of this particular situation, people with ostomies may be angry. Because anger results in the build-up and release of physical energy, it is important for you to learn how to cope with anger. Before you begin, it is first necessary to understand what anger is all about.

WHAT IS ANGER?

When you have a desire or goal in mind, and something interferes with your achievement of it, a feeling of tension and hostility may result from the developing frustration. This is what we refer to as anger. In Louise's case, her goal was to attend the party. She felt that her ostomy surgery thwarted those plans.

THREE TYPES OF ANGER

It can be helpful to discuss three different ways of experiencing anger. Rage is the expression of violent, uncontrolled anger. If Sandra was upset about her surgery, and a "friend" told her that surgery wouldn't have been necessary if she had taken better care of herself, you can imagine how angry she might be. Her rage might even lead her to say or do things that would certainly not enhance the prospects of a long-lasting, warm relationship with this person! Rage is probably the most intense anger you can experience. It is an outward expression of anger, as it results in a visible explosion. Rage can be a destructive release of the intense physical energy that builds up.

A second type of anger is resentment. This is the feeling of anger that is usually kept inside. What if Sandra listened to her friend's well-meaning comments, smiled and said nothing, but was seething inside? Resentment is a growing, smoldering feeling of anger directed towards a person or an object. However, it is kept bottled up. It tends to sit uncomfortably within you, and can create even more physiological and psychological damage.

The third type of anger is indignation. Indignation is considered the more appropriate, positive type of anger. It is released in a more controlled way. If Sandra had responded to the comments by stating that she appreciated her friend's concern, but she'd prefer no advice at this point or she might scream, this might have been a more appropriate response. Obviously, these three types of anger can occur in combination, or in different ways. However, understanding the different ways of experiencing anger can help you to cope with it more effectively.

Insults from other people, aside from everyday frustrations, can cause anger. "If you didn't eat all those prunes, you wouldn't have needed that terrible surgery!" This is not the kind of comment that will make you feel friendly! If you feel that someone is taking advantage of you, or you feel forced to do something that you do not want to do, anger may result. If you do not have the ability or confidence to say "no" when friends ask for a favor, this can create feelings of anger, especially when combined with the fact that you may not feel well.

In addition to the causes of anger mentioned above, there is one more. How about your ostomy as a cause of anger? Aren't you angry because you needed surgery? There may not be any specific reason you can point to. Or you might be able to list dozens of reasons. But being aware of this is important, because you must be aware of the anger to help yourself deal with it. Unfortunately, resolving your anger won't make your ostomy go away. Nor should you say that you'll only stop being angry when your ostomy is no longer needed. Neither attitude will help you. As we go on, we will be discussing ways of reducing anger and feeling better.

DOES YOUR MIND MAKE YOU ANGRY?

It is important to realize that anger exists uniquely in the mind of each angry individual. This anger is a direct result of your thoughts, rather than events. The event may lead to anger, but it is your interpretation of the event, the way you think or feel about it, which creates the anger. However, an event by itself does not produce anger. This is a very important point, one that will be discussed in much more detail a little bit later in the section, *Dealing With Anger*, so stay tuned!

ANGER AND YOUR BODY

When you are angry, a number of physiological responses occur in your body. Breathing becomes more rapid, blood pressure increases (you may feel like your blood is "boiling"), and your heart may begin to pound. Your face may get "hot," and your muscles become tense. You may feel stronger when angry. The more intense the anger is, the greater this feeling of power. I'm sure you can remember a time when you were so angry that you felt you had superhuman strength.

Anger is a form of energy. The more physical energy that builds up in the body due to anger, the more necessary it becomes for you to release it. The energy cannot be destroyed, so if it is not released in some constructive manner, it will eventually come out in another, less desirable way. Imagine the energy from anger as a stick of dynamite about to explode. If you get rid of it, it will explode away from you. It may cause some damage, but it will not hurt you inside as much as if you swallowed the dynamite to keep others from being hurt. Obviously, the ideal solution is not to throw the stick of dynamite, and not to swallow it, but (are you ready for this?) to try and de-fuse the dynamite! More about de-fusing soon.

Usually, extreme anger can pass quickly. If, however, the anger lasts for a long period of time, it can have physically damaging effects on the body. You've all heard about some of the physical problems that can result from holding in anger: ulcers, hypertension, headaches. It's just not good for your body.

When anger becomes extreme or turns into rage, you may feel like exploding. You may feel that, unless you are able to punch, kick, or hit something, and get rid of the anger in some way, you may lose control. Hopefully, this angry energy can be released without causing damage to another person, property, or yourself. If, when you finally calm down, you find that you have done something destructive, you may get angry at yourself all over again. Or you may feel another negative emotion, such as guilt.

ANGER AND YOUR MIND

Anger is usually experienced as an unpleasant feeling. However, this unpleasant feeling may exist along with a more pleasant feeling of power or strength. Frequently, the unpleasantness of anger is related to its consequences—knowing what you do when you are angry, and not being happy about it. If you lose control when you're angry, you'll probably even be afraid of it, and of what you might do next time!

DIFFERENT REACTIONS TO ANGER

Maureen, a 28-year-old teacher, was tired of her supervisor's pampering at work. Initially it was nice, but now she was ready to fulfill all her former responsibilities. Her supervisor, Mrs. Meeker, wouldn't let her do anything by herself. Let's see how this situation might be experienced in different ways.

The "Ignore" Approach

Because you feel like you may completely lose control, or feel overwhelmed by the intensity of your anger, you may try to do whatever you can to avoid the experience. This could include pushing thoughts out of your mind, even when you realize you are getting angry. Maureen might try to absorb herself in her activities, and ignore the fact that her supervisor is being so restrictive. She might try to agree with Mrs. Meeker that she shouldn't do as much. Although this might be upsetting, it could be temporarily effective in helping her to ignore the smothering. In the long run, however, you can see that this is not the best way to deal with anger.

The "Action" Approach

From another point of view, you might see anger as a necessary part of life, despite its unpleasantness. You know that there will be times when you'll be angry, whether you like it or not. You'll just have to deal with it as best you can.

In this case, Maureen would realize that she's not happy about being angry, and that she should firmly speak to her supervisor, to help her to understand more about her physical condition and what she can do. Hopefully, a better understanding can be reached, but at least Maureen knows that she's doing something about her feelings.

The "Power" Approach

Maybe you enjoy the flow of energy and strength that comes from being angry. Perhaps this is when you are best able to assert yourself to accomplish something. Here, Maureen knows that if she is pampered once too often she will explode. She loves the feeling of power that this anger gives her. She is almost looking forward to wiping the smile right off Mrs. Meeker's motherly face. If you enjoy this feeling, it is possible that you may even provoke situations to make yourself angry! An example of this would be professional football players or boxers, who psyche themselves up before a confrontation with an opponent. Becoming as angry as possible is the best preparation for a successful performance.

Your own reaction to anger is unique. It may also change from time to time. There may be times when you accept anger and almost value it as a motivator. At other times you may attempt to push this anger away.

Maureen might enjoy expressing her anger. But if her financial situation warned her not to chance losing her job, or if she really didn't want to hurt Mrs. Meeker, it might be better for her to have a calm discussion with her boss instead of exploding.

IS ANGER GOOD OR BAD?

How could anger possibly be good? Many people feel that nothing constructive can be gained from it. "Avoid anger at all costs because nothing good comes from it . . . Anger will get you into trouble, so don't let it happen." This is true, but only if you don't deal with the anger properly. Anger can be dangerous if it is kept inside. Remember that stick of dynamite? What an explosive example! If anger is released in destructive ways, it can cause problems in relationships (to say the least!). It can create physical problems as well, and can certainly aggravate your already-existing, ostomy-related problems. Does this mean that anger can make your condition worse? Well, what if you're so angry at somebody or something that you decide not to take care of yourself properly? For example, you don't take enough time to change your appliance, cleanse yourself, or properly irrigate. What if you're angry at someone who cares about you, and normally helps you with your appliance, or other aspects of your care? That person, if upset by your anger, may be less willing to help you. This may, in turn, make you feel even worse. So if you want your anger to be good instead of bad, try to turn it into something that can be helpful rather than harmful to you.

Anger *can* be constructive. It can mobilize your efforts and make you stronger to deal with an anger-provoking situation. Believe it or not, you might even handle a situation more successfully than you would if you weren't angry! Anger can give you a feeling of power or strength, of confidence or assertiveness. But don't get me wrong. I'm not saying that you should slam your finger with a hammer, or tell someone to punch you, in order to get yourself angry enough to solve all of your problems. What I am saying is that anger can be constructive, and it can help you to solve problems. Anger has two main benefits. First, it is an indicator that something is wrong. Something must be creating this feeling of anger—something that needs attention. Second, anger can motivate you to deal more actively with life's problems. You can become so emotionally charged that it will have a positive effect on your life.

In order for anger to be helpful, there are some very important things to keep in mind. First, don't let yourself become overwhelmed by the anger. Once that happens it is much harder for you to do what you have to do. Second, don't be afraid of your anger. If you do fear it, you will probably be unable to release it directly. More than likely, it will come out in unhealthy ways, or you will bottle it up inside. Third, be sure that the way you handle your anger is socially acceptable. Maureen might get a kick out of blowing up Mrs. Meeker's house, but would the police approve? Try to be flexible enough to recognize an appropriate way of releasing your anger.

DEALING WITH ANGER

You've already begun to realize that anger can be constructive. Hopefully, the information you've read so far has encouraged you in coping with anger. But what else can actually be done?

Because anger is such a complex emotion, and because so many things can lead to feelings of anger, there are no simple answers. Sorry about that! Does that mean that there is nothing that anybody can do about anger? No. Some things can be done to reduce the feelings of anger and allow them to be handled more efficiently, comfortably, and safely.

Step One—Admit that You're Angry

The first step in dealing with anger is to recognize that you are angry in the first place. As simple as this may sound, many people cannot even admit when they are angry. They may try to deny it, or rationalize their feelings that being angry is a sign of weakness. Therefore, since they don't want to feel weak, they won't admit that they are angry. They may feel that there is no appropriate reason for anger; therefore, they are acting in a childish way. But in order to work on anything in an attempt to change it, you've got to first admit that it exists.

How can you tell that you're angry if you're not sure? (Yes, there are some people who are not sure.) If you feel very tense (jumping at the sound of the telephone), or if you find yourself reacting impulsively (slamming down the phone when you get a wrong number and storming out of the house) or with hostility (cursing at your neighbor for leaving a smidgeon of garbage on your lawn), chances are that you're angry. Remember: until you recognize that you are angry, you cannot do anything constructive about it.

Step Two—Where does your Anger Come From?

The second step in dealing with anger is trying to identify its source. Where does it come from? What is contributing to it? What events have led to these feelings of anger? Why do you want to put your fist through a wall? For one thing, your surgery may lead to anger. You may be angry with yourself for neglecting your condition. You may feel anger towards your physician, whether justified or not. You may be angry because you've lost bowel control. You may be angry because of the extra time involved in changing appliances, or because of added costs. You may be angry at your surgeon for creating the ostomy that has marred your once blemish-free abdomen!

In some cases, the events leading to anger may be quite obvious. In cases, however, the source of anger may be vague and unclear. It may be hard to pinpoint what is causing it. At such times, you should try to probe even more deeply to come up with possible causes of your anger.

Of course, much of this anger is irrational. But, like other emotional reactions, it must be worked through. It cannot just be pushed away. Simply telling yourself, "don't be angry," is not enough. You must learn to channel it more effectively.

Guilt can sometimes confuse you if you are trying to identify the source of anger. Josie was a 32-year-old mother of three. She woke up one morning, went downstairs and found her kitchen a disaster area. Taking care of the kitchen was a responsibility that she had given to her children, because she was physically unable to handle it during her recovery from surgery. She found herself screaming at them for not fulfilling their responsibilities. In actuality, however, her anger may have been a reflection, not of hostility towards her children, but of guilt about her own inability to handle her kitchen responsibilities.

Step Three—Why are you Angry?

It is now necessary to explain to yourself why you are angry. In Josie's case, she could explain her anger by her inability to do what she wanted to do. Josie wanted to be able to fulfill her responsibilities as a mother and housewife. She felt that taking care of the kitchen was included in this. Because she was unable to do so, and did not have enough physical strength, she felt angry.

Why is this step important? Mainly, to decide whether or not the anger that you are feeling is realistic. Analyze your reasons for being angry. If you recognize that your reasons are not realistic, this alone can help you to deal with these feelings of anger. If, on the other hand, you can objectively say that your feelings of anger are realistic, then the next step is to decide how you are going to deal with them properly.

How do you deal with them properly? You have already begun! By working through the first three steps, you have received information that will be very helpful in your efforts to deal with your anger.

THOUGHTS CAN MAKE YOU ANGRY

In the past, it was falsely believed that there were only two possible ways to deal with anger: to keep it inside, or to let it out.

But what about a third possibility? Remember before when we talked about de-fusing that stick of dynamite? Our anger is a result of the way we think! In our minds, we are actually interpreting those events that lead to anger. If we can change the way we interpret events, and reorganize our thinking patterns, is it possible to stop creating the anger that we feel? Of course! We can learn to control our thoughts *before* they make us angry, regardless of what the events were. Ask yourself this question: if something happened that made you angry, would everybody in the world be angry because of it? No. The reason why you are angry is because that's the way you think about or interpret the event. Other people aren't angry because they did not interpret the event in a way that made them so. For example, let's say you've made a doctor's appointment. Ten minutes before you were ready to leave, his nurse called to cancel, saying he'd reschedule the appointment at another time. You might be furious, because you felt you should have received more notice, and because you really wanted to see him. "Who does he think he is?" But others might not interpret it that way, and might not get the least bit angry. So if we can learn to interpret events in a more positive, constructive, and calm manner, we can reduce feelings of anger. We wouldn't have to decide whether we wanted to let anger out or keep it inside because, by controlling our thoughts, anger would not even exist most of the time.

You have already completed one of the four steps in reorganizing your thoughts to prevent anger. You have learned that anger can be good and constructive. It can help you to solve problems, and you don't have to be afraid of it. Just becoming aware of its positive elements can help you to be less afraid of anger. This can help you to deal with the thoughts that may make you angry.

GOOD ANGRY THOUGHTS VS. BAD ANGRY THOUGHTS

Writing down what you think is making you angry can be very helpful. Good angry thoughts can move you to positive, constructive action. You might want to plan your strategies for resolving the problem. On the other hand, many of your thoughts may include so much anger, and be so destructive, that you feel like banging your head against the wall. Be honest when writing down your thoughts, regardless of how violent or profane they may be. Such rich, colorful language can be helpful in getting your feelings out and down on paper. This will ultimately help you to control your anger. Try to look at these thoughts more objectively, the way someone else might look at them. Attempt to bring them down to a more manageable level.

MENTAL MOVIES

An interesting technique that can be helpful in controlling anger is imagery, or "watching movies in your mind." When you become angry, you frequently have all kinds of pictures in your head of what is making you angry and what you'd like to do to deal with it. These movies can be very helpful.

For example, imagine that you are very, very tired. Your friend calls to tell you that her car has broken down. Could you please pick up her dry-cleaning? When you tell her that you are too tired to go, she says something about how she can never depend on you for anything. This is a friend? You are furious. At that moment, imagine all the abusive things that you would like to say to her, and imagine the shocked expression on her face. If you ask her to hold on for a moment, and close your eyes and imagine this as if you were actually doing it, you'll probably be able to complete the phone call without destroying a friendship. You should feel relieved of much of your anger. You may even smile or laugh as you think about the scenes that are playing through your mind. More about imagery in the chapter, *Pain*.

Nora was quite fed up with her son, Pesty Pete. Whenever she asked for his help with normal household chores, his answers were fresh and abusive. Just before she was about to give him a haircut with a meat cleaver, she remembered the mental movie technique. She imagined herself strangling him—his eyeballs popping and gurgling sounds coming from his throat. This helped to get rid of the intense, angry feelings that were making her crazy, and allowed her to deal with Pete more constructively. (No, she's not in jail.)

THE BIG, RED STOP SIGN

Another technique that can help you to control anger is referred to as "thought stopping." Remember: it is the thoughts in your mind that are making you angry. These are the thoughts you have upon interpreting an event. When you find that angry thoughts have come into your head, picture a big red stop sign. Seeing that word in your mind will serve as a momentary distraction. Then concentrate on something you enjoy, whether it is a type of food, an activity, or a movie or television program. Whatever you choose, you will divert your thinking, and have a better chance of dissipating your anger. You could also participate in a pleasant distracting activity, such as reading a book, taking a walk, or calling a friend, which will also help you to feel less angry.

CHANGE YOUR REQUIREMENTS

People often get angry when they want certain things to occur in certain ways. When your specific requirements are not met, you may feel angry. Trying to modify your requirements can help you to cope with anger.

Let's say that you're not feeling well and you decide to call your doctor. His answering service tells you that he is not in—he will call back within a half-hour. After 45 minutes, when he has still not returned your call, you are fuming. Why? Because your requirement that he call back within 30 minutes has not been met. Revise your requirement. Tell yourself that you would have liked him to call back within 30 minutes, but he may be tied up in some way. You'll be satisfied if he calls you at his earliest convenience. By modifying the requirement, you can feel less angry.

Another way to benefit from this technique is to write down those thoughts indicating what your requirements are. Then try to write down new, more flexible desires. This will make you feel much better.

PUT YOURSELF IN THEIR SHOES

One of the best ways of dealing with anger towards somebody else is to try to understand exactly what that person is feeling: what the person wants, why the person is saying what he or she is saying. This will make you more aware of why somebody else is behaving or talking the way he or she is and you will be better able to deal with it constructively. This will also help you to understand what the other person will feel if he or she is the target of your abusive release of anger.

LET IT OUT LESS EXPLOSIVELY

We have discussed a number of ways to control your thinking and improve your ability to interpret events in ways that will prevent anger. But what if this doesn't always work? It is new for some of you and requires effort. What if there are times when you find yourself angrier than ever? What can be done to deal with anger constructively when it already exists?

TALK, DON'T BITE

Obviously, it is much more desirable to have a constructive discussion over an issue than an angry exchange of heated words, which accomplishes nothing. In most cases, anger arises from a conflict or problem with another person; therefore, it is frequently helpful to improve your ability to get your point across constructively. You are trying to negotiate a better resolution to a problem that may exist between you and somebody else. A heated argument, or "fighting fire with fire," is not the answer. Instead, you want to fight the fire by dousing it—reducing the heatedness of the argument. Try complimenting the person or looking for the positive things in what that person is saying to you, even if you're angry. This works in two ways. One, it will probably surprise the person. Two, you will be focusing on words or thoughts that are more constructive, rather than letting yourself get angry because of what's being said. Calmly restate your feelings.

HOW ABOUT PHYSICAL ACTIVITY?

In general, one of the best outlets for releasing angry energy is physical activity. If you are a new ostomate and haven't yet recovered all of your energy, this outlet may not be available. Interestingly, it has been found that physical energy from anger can be released by watching things. For example, by watching a sporting event, you aren't releasing energy through participation in the sport, but you may still be able to "get into it" and reduce your anger that way. Or try watching a particularly violent or emotionally draining movie. You can become so totally absorbed that the energy building up from anger is released through worry, fear, or excitement. A movie or book that allows you to identify with the characters, or where the characters allow release of anger, can be beneficial as well. A common outlet for anger, especially among children, is crying. Crying has long been considered very effective. I'm sure you've heard of the therapeutic effects of a good cry. However, this technique is not for everyone. People who can be more open in expressing their emotions may be better able to benefit from this outlet.

Some people like to count to ten when angry. This can distract you from what is making you angry, giving you a chance to calm down and think about it more constructively. Try counting to a thousand, if necessary!

LET US REVIEW

It is very important to remember that events alone do not make you angry. It is your thoughts, your interpretations of these events, that lead to anger. Even if something really terrible happens, it is the meaning that you give to this particular event that makes you angry. It is the way you think about this terrible event that creates your anger. Since your thinking makes you angry, *you* are responsible for feeling this way. Therefore, you can be just as responsible for changing your thinking to help yourself cope with anger, or at least reducing it to a more manageable level.

The best way to handle anger is probably to be in control enough so that it doesn't build up in the first place. But if it does, remember that anger does have its benefits. However, it only has benefits if it is channeled and used constructively. In general, uncontrolled anger is an unpleasant, negative, and destructive emotion. Your efforts are best spent in trying to figure out how to reorganize your thinking so that it doesn't get out of hand.

11

Guilt

Have you ever felt guilty? Many ostomates say that they have. Guilt is a very unpleasant emotion. Let's take a look at what leads to guilty feelings.

THE TWO COMPONENTS OF GUILT

Feelings of guilt usually have two components. The first of these is the "wrongdoing;" you feel that you have either done something wrong, or haven't done something that you should have done. The second component is the "self-blame;" you blame yourself for doing this wrong thing, and feel that you are "bad" because of it. That's the culprit! It is the concept of "badness" that creates the guilty feeling. If you feel bad about doing something wrong, this is normal and understandable. But when you start telling yourself that you are bad, guilt follows. What if other people tell you that "it's o.k.?" This may not help. Your feeling of guilt may have nothing to do with what others tell you or what they think. Even if they disagree with you, these are still your feelings. Remember: your guilt comes from the feeling that you are a bad person, rather than from feeling bad about what you have done. Is it fitting to label yourself as a bad person or blame yourself because you've done something wrong? Even if you have done something wrong, it's better to label that particular behavior as bad, rather than yourself.

Is the behavior that you are blaming yourself for really that terrible or wrong? Does it justify the feeling of badness that leads to guilt?

WHAT IS VS. WHAT OUGHT TO BE

Do you see a difference between the way you are doing something and the way you think you should be doing it? If so, you can really feel the old guilt horns! How do you work this out? Major union/management problems would be easier to solve! Can you work harder or do more? If you can, then do it. If not, try examining your day-to-day goals for working and living. Check to see if these goals are practical, considering what you can and cannot do because of your ostomy. Try to take more pride in what you *can* do. Although most people hate hearing, "things could be worse," this phrase is quite true. You might not be able to do anything at all. If you concentrate on the things you can do, and place less emphasis on what you can't, your feelings of guilt will diminish. You'll feel a lot better. Changing the emphasis in your thinking will also help you to lessen the gap between what is and what ought to be. This is what led to these guilty feelings in the first place.

TALK IT OVER

It is very important to discuss how you feel about your condition with others who may be affected by it. It is helpful to talk over feelings with the important people in your life, to share concerns, and try to figure out solutions to problems. Maryanne, a 22-year-old woman who had been married under a year, had enjoyed a very active social life before developing symptoms leading to ostomy surgery. In addition to going out on weekends, she and her husband would go out with friends or participate in other social activities at least two or three evenings during the week. Now, because of her concern with her ostomy, she refused to go out as frequently. Somtimes, she wouldn't want to go out at all during an entire week. Not only did she feel unhappy about her condition, but she felt extremely guilty at holding her husband back. She felt that he couldn't have a good time because of her. It would be helpful for Maryanne to discuss alternatives with her husband. Maryanne should work on her fears and try to reduce her reluctance to go out. Techniques discussed in the chapter, *Fears and Anxieties*, could be very helpful. As Maryanne became less concerned about and less sensitive to her ostomy, she'd probably be more willing to socialize, either at home or out. Arriving at a solution, with her husband's cooperation, could effectively reduce guilt feelings and improve the marriage.

So far, we have been discussing how doing the wrong thing can lead to guilt. But it's not "behavioral mistakes" alone that lead to guilty feelings. Thoughts can also become upsetting enough to result in guilt.

THOUGHTS CAN HURT, TOO

Sometimes, you may feel guilty without doing anything wrong. You may be merely thinking things that cause guilt. Marlene, a 29-year-old woman with two children, said that she felt guilty because her 58-year-old mother was spending so much time taking care of her and her kids. Marlene felt guilty because she was still so weak. She asked how long her mother would have to take care of her. The fact that her father complained about not having enough time with her mother didn't help matters any, either. Should Marlene blame herself and feel guilty because of her condition, something she could not control? Since she hadn't really done anything wrong, Marlene could feel better by modifying her thinking.

In order to successfully cope with guilt, you must first focus on what led to the guilty feelings. Have you actually done something wrong? Have you really neglected something you shouldn't have? You may feel guilty about your thoughts or desires, rather than specific actions or behaviors. Recognize that, if you haven't done anything to lead to guilt, then you should identify those thoughts that are making you feel like a bad person. If you can learn to talk to yourself in a positive way, looking at your thoughts objectively and constructively, guilt can be reduced.

Frequently, as in Marlene's case, feeling guilty is related to seeing yourself as responsible for others' actions or behaviors. The more responsible you feel, the more guilt you may feel, especially if you cannot fulfill your responsibility. In dealing with this, it is important to be able to explain why you feel this responsibility. Frequently, just asking the question "why?" will point out that this thinking is unrealistic. That alone can help to reduce guilt. This is another reason why discussions with other important people are helpful. They may explain why taking the responsibility for someone else is inappropriate. Be sure to place feelings of responsibility in proper perspective. There is a limit as to how responsible you should feel for others' actions or feelings—they are responsible for their own. Nor are you responsible for having an ostomy, and for any restrictions this may place on you. Marlene should recognize that nobody was forcing her mother to take care of her or her children. Her mother chose this course of action. Marlene would have less guilt if she didn't feel responsible for her mother's choice. She might even begin to enjoy her mother's care. When individuals are not forced into an activity, they participate out of choice and desire. The same holds true for this book. You *are* reading it out of choice and desire, aren't you?

As another example of guilty thoughts, let's take a quick look at Linda. Linda was in a lot of pain, and had many questions about the condition of her stoma. However, she refused to call her doctor because of astronomical medical fees. You see, Linda felt guilty about the amount of money her husband had to shell out to doctors and surgeons. However, Linda must learn that this can't be helped. This doesn't make her a bad person. Things would be even worse if she didn't go to the doctor and her condition deteriorated!

"SHOULD" THOUGHTS

Among the most common causes of guilt are thoughts containing the word "should." Examples of such thoughts are, "I should have been able to finish that job today . . . We should have that party; all our friends have entertained us this year . . . You should have let me do the dishes . . . I shouldn't have any more pain." These "should" thoughts imply that you must be just about perfect, and on top of everything. When there is a difference between what you feel should occur and what actually does occur, guilt can result. You will become upset whenever you fall short of your "should." Should thoughts lead to guilt simply because they are not sensible, realistic, or justifiable? Should you blame yourself because they set up goals that you may not be able to fulfill?

Now that I've explained what you shouldn't do, what exactly should you do? In order to feel better and reduce feelings of guilt, it is helpful to reword your thoughts to eliminate "should" thoughts. Try to use less demanding words. Say, "It would be nice if I could finish that job today, but I can't," rather than, "I should finish that job today." If your physical condition forces you to stay in bed, you'll feel much more guilty when "should" thoughts remind you of unfulfilled obligations. If you have trouble changing the wording of your "should" thoughts, try asking yourself, "Why should I . . . ?" or "Who says I should . . . ?" or "Where is it written that I should . . . ?" This may help you decide whether you are setting up impossible requirements for yourself. It can also help you to reduce your feelings of guilt.

Let's say, for example, that you are thinking of having a party because all your friends have invited you to get-togethers. Ask yourself why you should. Is it because the "Party Rulebook" tells you that, if you don't have a party, your friendship license will be revoked? Is it because, if you don't have a party, your friends (some friends!) won't invite you to their homes anymore? If you can think of realistic answers to these questions, it will be easier to realize that you don't have to have a party. Although it would be nice, it is more acceptable to wait until you feel better.

THE CONSEQUENCES OF GUILT

So far, we've been discussing what leads to guilt, how you may feel, and how you can try to adjust your thoughts and behaviors to feel better. But what happens if you have not yet been successful in eliminating guilt? People who feel guilty frequently act in negative ways to hide from these feelings. There may be a tendency to indulge in "escape" behaviors, such as drinking or excessive sleeping, which do not deal with problems head-on but, instead, attempt to push them away.

Anna, a 24-year-old receptionist, felt guilty because she had stopped making plans with her friends. The reason: she was still embarrassed about her ostomy. As a result, she began to lose friends, and her guilt became more and more difficult to bear. She began drinking after work, and going to bed right after dinner, in an attempt to forget her misery. This behavior did not help the situation any. Instead, it compounded the problem. Now Anna had something else to feel guilty about: her escape behavior. This could increase the feeling of badness, leading to even more guilt and creating a vicious cycle. The first step towards improvement is to look past the escape behavior and identify whatever is causing the guilt.

Consider what can be done to rectify the problem causing the guilt. At the same time, try to eliminate the escape behaviors, recognizing that they are only a cop-out. It is possible, however, for there to be no clear-cut solution to the events or feelings creating guilt. If, for example, Anna's ostomy is keeping her from making plans with her friends, can she believe that the only way to make things better is for her ostomy to go away? This would certainly be wishful thinking! Don't give up because no complete solutions exist. Look for partial solutions, which can still help to reduce guilt by reminding you that you are trying to improve the situation. Anna's ostomy won't go away, but she could try to reduce her reluctance to get together with friends. Again, if fear of leakage, odor, or other things contribute to this reluctance, be sure to read the chapter, *Fears and Anxieties*.

OTHER SUGGESTIONS

We've talked a lot about how thoughts and behaviors can cause guilt. But what if you just feel guilty and can't remember what you were thinking or doing to make you feel that way? How can you start using all these great thought-changing ideas if you don't remember what thoughts you want to change? Good question! In order to identify those thoughts or behaviors that directly or indirectly lead to guilt, it is frequently helpful to keep a brief, written log of feelings or activities that may have caused your guilt. Once you have written these things down, you can then begin figuring out how to change them, improving your outlook, and reducing your guilt.

Alice, age 37, had been feeling increasingly guilty since her surgery but didn't really know why. By keeping a log, she noticed that she had been arriving at work late on a regular basis. She wasn't aware of how frequently she had been late, and she had always been proud of her punctuality. The log helped her to see that she must improve her morning routine in order to be more punctual. As she worked on this problem, her guilt lessened.

What about those negative thoughts that lead to guilt? It can be very helpful to try and turn these thoughts around, making them more positive and guilt-free. For example, let's say that you feel guilty because you believe you are a bad parent. Ask yourself if you have ever done anything that a good parent might do. Just about every parent can come up with something. Here begins the process of eliminating your "bad parent blues." The idea is to turn your mind's negative thoughts into reasonable, positive ones. This way, the feeling of guilt will not take a strangle-hold!

A FINAL GUILTY THOUGHT

Guilt is a very destructive emotion, one that can present major obstacles to your success in coping with your ostomy. By becoming aware of how guilt develops, you have a much better chance of effectively employing coping strategies to reduce guilt and its negative effects.

12

Stress

What is stress? Stress is a response that occurs in your body. It helps you mobilize your strength to deal with different things happening in your life. Many things occur each day that require you to adapt. These are the "stressors." All the changes that occur in your body when something (the stressor) provokes you are called stress responses.

IS STRESS GOOD OR BAD?

A certain amount of stress is normal—and necessary. Stress helps you to "get your act together," and prepares you to handle your life in the best possible way. Now you're probably thinking, "So why do I always hear people talking about how stress can be harmful?" When people talk about the harmful effects of stress, they are referring to situations where there is *too much* stress. Then it can become destructive. If left unchecked, it can eat away at you and drain all of your energy.

Elaine, a 35-year-old housewife, was under pressure. Her husband was bringing his boss home for dinner. She was still weak from surgery, and was pacing herself in preparing the meal so she wouldn't get run down. The stress she felt was tolerable; that is, until the phone rang. Her husband called, telling her that, due to an emergency business meeting that evening, they'd be arriving two hours early! Elaine's stress was no longer tolerable!

Reasonable amounts of stress can be handled. They can even be helpful. In this chapter, however, we'll be talking about harmful stress. This is the type that can hurt if not controlled.

The word "stress" is used very frequently these days. It's used to refer to things that create nervousness, anxiety, tension, anger, or an upset feeling. These are all actually parts of stress, rather than the same thing. In other words, they may cause the stress response.

WHO FEELS STRESS?

Everyone experiences stress. Nobody escapes it. But since stress can be positive or negative, learning how to respond positively will lead to a more successful emotional and physical life. If you have a hard time responding to stress, this won't be easy. Some people are more vulnerable to negative stress responses than others. Are you?

THE STRESS RESPONSE

Every person has a unique way of responding to stress. Stress control (controlling how you respond to stress) is within your reach. Your pattern of response depends on a number of things—your upbringing, self-esteem, beliefs about yourself and the world, what you say to yourself, and how you guide yourself in your actions and thoughts. The degree to which you feel in control of your life plays a role in your stress response. The way you feel physically and emotionally, and the way you get along with people, are also a part of it. To sum it up, everyone's method of dealing with stress is unique and individual, and depends on a complex combination of thoughts and behaviors.

Stressor + Interpretation = Stress Response

The way that we respond to stress depends on the chemistry between two factors. The first factor is the stressor, or the outside pressures. What is going on around you that is creating the reactions? The second factor is what is within you, or how you interpret things. It is the interaction of the stimulus and your own internal reaction that determines your response to stress. This has important implications for coping with stress, when you realize that it is not just the environment that causes your response, but also the way you interpret the stressor. Some stressors in the environment would produce stress in anybody. What would happen, for example, if somebody pointed a knife at your throat? Calm acceptance, or a stress response? Get the point? It's important to learn how to reduce the number of stressors that negatively affect you, and improve your reaction to those you can't avoid.

BODY VS. MIND

How do you respond to stress? Like one's response to anger or other mobilizing emotions, there are two main ways: physically and cognitively. A cognitive response includes the way you think and feel. Most people respond to stress in both ways, although it is possible for you to respond in only one way.

What happens physically? If you experience a stressful situation, the circulatory system speeds up. Blood is pushed rapidly towards different parts of the body, particularly those parts necessary to protect you. Because the blood supply is diverted towards these essential parts, the supply to the digestive system is usually reduced. As a result, the digestive process slows down, making it work less efficiently.

Chronic or prolonged stress puts a severe strain on your body. When strong, your body can fight off most foreign invaders, bacteria, and germs. As a result, many diseases can be avoided. But prolonged stress puts such a strain on the body that your defense mechanisms may break down. This, in turn, makes your body more vulnerable to the very problems you'd like to avoid!

As an ostomate, you may be even more aware of the effects of physiological stress. Not only does stress cause changes in the digestive system, but urinary or fecal output may be changed as well. Because you are so much more aware of your elimination process, you may be able to recognize a change and benefit from stress management.

Have you heard of the "fight or flight" syndrome? Animals do this when they feel threatened. The animal prepares either to fight or run away, a purely physical response. You will not see an animal standing there, scratching his head, and thinking about what should be done! But humans have the unique ability to think and reason! Lucky us! So we include cognitive responses in our repertoire. By the way, researchers feel that this is one of the main reasons why human beings are susceptible to so much stress-related physical illness. By thinking, instead of acting, we may not be dealing with stress as effectively as we might.

When does stress lead to physical problems? When you can't respond to stress in a way that eliminates it, the stress continues unabated. Being unable to do anything about it may cause even more stress, creating a vicious cycle. This can take its toll on your body.

You may be vulnerable to stress in your own unique way. Certain parts of your body may tend to be more vulnerable and, when stressors occur, it is these parts that feel the effect. For example, have you ever felt extreme intestinal discomfort and automatically clutched your stomach because of stress? Or have you ever endured a painful headache? Stress may have even played a role in the illness or condition leading to your surgery. Isn't that marvelous?

What happens if you respond to stress physically? You may tremble or perspire. Your face may flush. You may feel a surge of adrenaline flowing through your body. Your mouth may become dry or you may feel nauseous. Your breathing may become more rapid and shallow. Your heart may begin to pound. Your muscles become tight, creating headaches, cramps, or other painful reactions. Sounds lovely, doesn't it?

Your cognitive or emotional response to stress may not be as visible. You won't be able to concentrate as well. Your attention span may be reduced. You may have trouble learning something new. You may be afraid to do things. You may withdraw or feel nervous. You may lose confidence in yourself. You'll become aware of any unpleasant physical responses, and these may make you feel even more stressed. For example, if you feel stress and respond with shallow, rapid breathing or heart palpitations, being aware of these physical responses may create even more stress. This can lead to feelings of panic.

THREE RESPONSES TO STRESS

When a stressful stimulus occurs, you will most likely respond in one of three ways. You might respond immediately and impulsively without giving enough thought to a better response. You might not respond at all, and either try to ride it out, or become so frozen that you are unable to respond. Finally, you may respond to stressors in a well-planned, organized, and effective manner. If so, you may not even need this chapter! But if not, read on!

HOW TO DEAL WITH STRESS

Remember: stress can be managed and controlled, but it cannot be eliminated. Stress will always exist. You can deal with the amount of stress you endure and how intense that stress may be, but you'll never be able to make it go away. For a person who has had ostomy surgery, it is especially important that stress be controlled.

Let's begin by mentioning the wrong ways of responding to stress. These are the ways that *don't* help you: smoking, getting drunk, using drugs, overeating, and overactivity. These will merely distract you or else delay the effects of stress.

So what should you do? Try to learn new, more appropriate ways of dealing with stress than the methods you've been using.

Relaxation Procedures

The best way to start controlling stress is by using relaxation procedures. Try the "quick release" method discussed in the introductory chapter of this section. Other successful methods of relaxation include meditation, self-hypnosis, imagery, or even a warm bath! Deep breathing alone can help to eliminate tension from the body, slow down the heart, and create a better sense of well-being. Learning to relax can be helpful in reducing the amount of stress you are experiencing. It will give your body a chance to rest and recuperate as well. A stronger body can deal more effectively with the ranges of stress (or of life)!

Pinpointing Stressors

Stress is a type of energy that needs release. It can be handled either positively or negatively. Stress is negative when you cannot handle it well.

In order to learn how to cope successfully, you must first identify your stressors. What, specifically, is causing you to feel stress? Maybe it's a concern about leakage or odor. Maybe it's the pressure of a dissolving relationship. Maybe it's ongoing skin irritation. These are all possible ostomy-related stressors.

What if you're not sure what's causing it? How can you figure out what it is? One way is to keep a record of your activities and experiences, using numerical ratings, such as a scale called the SUD Scale. SUD stands for Subjective Units of Disturbance. How does it work? Ratings on this scale range from 0 to 100, depending on the amount of stress you are experiencing. Use 100 to represent the most extreme and disturbing stress, and 0 to represent no stress (total and complete relaxation). Then rate your activities and experiences on the SUD scale. The ones with the higher SUD numbers are the ones causing you the most stress. Now you're ready to move on.

Identify your Stress Reactions

Once you have begun identifying your stressors, you must then become completely aware of your responses to them. Are they more physiological or psychological? What parts of your body seem to be most vulnerable? What kind of reactions does your body show? Does your attention span suffer? Do you start losing confidence, or feel like you're slipping? As you become more aware of this, you will develop a more complete picture of your unique stress response. You will be able to recognize the stressors that affect you and how you react to them. You'll then be better able to decide whether or not you should modify your behavior in responding to the stressor.

What's the next step? Once you recognize which stressors are negative, try to determine whether or not you can eliminate them. If you can, start figuring out how to do it. Removing the source of stress is an obvious and logical way to manage stress. Develop a plan of attack. This might include a number of alternate strategies, all designed to remove or minimize the impact of the stressor. But, on the other hand, if you realize that you can't eliminate the source of your stress, you'll then have to work on your means of interpreting what's going on. You'll have to work on your thinking, and your responding, in order to manage stress. In such cases, changing the stressor is out of your control, but changing the way you react isn't. You might want to use some of the suggestions discussed in the chapters, *Depression* and *Anger*. The use of *systematic desensitization*, discussed in the chapter, *Fears and Anxieties*, can also be beneficial. Many techniques for changing your thinking have already been discussed in previous chapters.

Certain physical activities can be great for stress control. For example, some people can relieve tension or stress by driving. As long as the driver continues to observe safety rules, driving can be relaxing.

Exercise

Another important way of dealing with stress is by exercising. Fortunately, although you have experienced a major body change, you should soon be able to do practically any type of exercise you want to do. Therefore, exercise can be a much more practical method of stress control than it might be for other chronic conditions, where body movement is restricted or disabled. Virtually any type of exercise can be effective. Anything that gets the body moving, gets the heart pumping faster, and allows for a release of tension, is ideal.

Keeping Busy—The Fun Way

Hobbies or other leisure activities can be very helpful. They can divert your attention away from the stressful situation, directing it towards something more enjoyable. These activities will also help you feel productive. A lack of productivity may be one of the stressors giving you problems in the first place!

Another technique for dealing with stress is sleep. Some people have difficulty sleeping when experiencing high levels of stress. However, cat naps, short naps, or even prolonged periods of sleep may be possible and can help stress.

IN CONCLUSION

What are your goals? If stress is interfering with your achievement of these goals, then your stress response is negative. Learning how to control stress is a very necessary part of successfully achieving your goals, as well as successfully coping with your ostomy.

13

Other Emotions

The emotions we've covered so far in this section are not the only ones, of course. Worry, for example, is a basic emotion. What might you worry about? Have you got a month to discuss all possible worries? You've probably worried about the future, what your life will be like, what sexual activity will be like, how life will change because of the ostomy, among countless other things. What other emotions enter into the picture? This chapter will discuss four other emotions common in life with an ostomy: boredom, envy, grief, and upset.

BOREDOM

Hopefully, by this time, you are not so bored that you have stopped reading! As long as you aren't bored, let's talk a little about boredom! What an empty feeling! It's one of the worst feelings anyone can experience. It has been said that more problems and serious tragedies come from being bored than from any other single condition.

Why are you bored? There may be no meaningful activity going on, no stimulation or excitement. Your life may seem to be going nowhere. Nothing is challenging you, and there's no incentive to do anything. Because you weren't born bored, you must have learned to be bored. You weren't always bored, and even now you are not always bored. There are still certain things that keep your attention from time to time. Right?

"Unboring" Yourself

What can you do about it? The first step is to analyze why you are bored. What is causing the boredom? Obviously, figuring this out will help you to determine how you can improve things. Then you'll want to see what you can do to add some interest to your life. But don't feel that you must push yourself to enjoy something. Forcing yourself to become amused rarely works. You may find that activities you used to enjoy have become artificial and uninteresting. You no longer get any pleasure from them. That doesn't mean, however, that you shouldn't try to do anything. You do want to try some new activities that will make your life more interesting. Don't limit yourself to those things that used to interest you. Preferences change. Try things that never interested you before, because maybe now they will spark an interest in you.

Learn Something New!

One of the most effective weapons against boredom is learning. The mind is like a sponge, always ready and willing to soak up more information and knowledge. Select a potentially interesting topic you don't know much about. Try to learn something about it. You may want to begin by simply going to the library and reading some books on the topic. Maybe you'd like to enroll in an adult education course. Often, boredom quickly disappears once you are involved in something new. Learning is a great way to do this.

Is an Ostomy Boring?

I bet you never thought of an ostomy as boring. But it can be, primarily because of any restrictions you may have while you heal from surgery. Many activities that provide enjoyment for you may be temporarily out of reach. You may not even want to bother starting something new, not knowing how long it will be until you're back on your feet.

Mona, three weeks following ileostomy surgery, was too tired to leave her house. She couldn't go shopping or meet friends for lunch, and she was fed up with the garbage on television. Was Mona bored? You bet she was! A friend suggested that they play a new board game, since Mona had always enjoyed them. But she decided not to, since she didn't want to stop in the middle and attend to her appliance. So what do you do? Don't let your ostomy cause you to give up on life. Continue under the assumption that you will be able to do most of what you would like to do. If you do have to curtail any activities because of your condition, you'll do so. If you have to drop an activity, you'll drop it. But you don't have to eliminate everything from your life simply because you feel you won't complete them.

You can also become bored if your social life is not the greatest. What can you do about this? Once again, try to learn something, especially by taking courses of some kind. Aside from the mental stimulation you'll get from learning activities, you will also meet some stimulating and challenging people. Increasing your circle of friends is a good way to fight boredom.

Anticipation

One of the best ways to fight boredom is to always give yourself something to look forward to. It doesn't matter how small this may be. It can be as simple as reading a chapter of a good book, writing a letter, making that phone call you've been looking forward to, watching a television program you've been excited about, or meeting somebody special for lunch. Try to schedule something to look forward to every day. This way, even if part of your day seems boring, whether you're doing menial chores or just resting to build up your strength, you will at least have something enjoyable to look forward to. You won't give the weeds of boredom a chance to take root!

Goal-Setting

Set goals for yourself, both short-term and long-term. Boredom can arise from plodding along with no purpose in life. Having something specific and tangible to shoot for can be helpful in fighting boredom. This doesn't mean you'll never be bored. You may still have to give yourself a kick in the derriere occasionally to keep moving towards those goals. But isn't it better to have something to shoot for than to have nothing at all?

ENVY

You've heard the cliche, "the grass is always greener . . . " If you have an ostomy, you are probably envious of others who do not. This is understandable. You may even be envious of other people who can simply go to the bathroom!

Envy can be a destructive emotion, because it's a type of self-torture. It can be very painful. You're constantly putting yourself down and comparing yourself with the better qualities of somebody else. You feel inferior. This can lead to other feelings as well, such as anger or depression.

Why is envy a problem? Because it shows that you are not satisfied with being yourself. You want to be like somebody else. You want to have what somebody else has (or hasn't!). Does this mean that the other person has a happy life? Is that person happier than you in every way? You may have an ostomy, but this doesn't mean that everything else about the other person's life is superior. Stop and think for a moment. I'm sure you can come up with some areas in which your life is better!

Is Envy a Positive Emotion?

In general, emotions usually serve a purpose. Emotions such as anger and anxiety mobilize you to prepare to handle their sources. On the other hand, envy is a destructive emotion. It does not have the positive qualities that other emotions may have. But don't just throw in your wet handkerchief. If your recognize that you're envious, analyze the reason why. Try to change this by concentrating on yourself and your own attributes. Don't let envy get you down.

How Does Envy Occur?

Basically, there are four conditions necessary for you to feel envy. First, you feel deprived. You feel like you can't have something that you want or need. This doesn't just mean money or pleasure. Envy is an intense feeling that involves more than this. It seems like your feeling of need lies deep inside. Second, somebody else has whatever it is that you feel you're missing. Third, you feel powerless to do anything about it. You feel totally unable to change the circumstances that have made you envious in the first place. This helplessness causes you to feel more and more bitter. This makes you even more envious! Fourth, there is a change in the relationship between you and whatever it is that you envy, be it person, object, or situation. You no longer simply compare yourself with the other, but feel fiercely competitive. You may begin to feel that the only reason you don't have what you would like is because somebody else does.

If you feel envious, is it necessarily the same kind of envy that everyone feels? No. There are actually two types of envy. One is an envy of tangible things (cars, boats, homes, friends, and so on). The other is less tangible. If you have an ostomy, you may still have many tangible things. You may still have a family, a car, and a place to live. You may still have a job. But the fact that you can't enjoy these things as much as somebody else can make you envious, and this is more emotional.

What Can You Do?

Concentrate on being yourself. Increase the positive benefits and enjoyments you can get out of life. Why worry about comparing yourself with somebody else? What's that going to do? Sure, you may not have the same body parts as you did before surgery. This may have other implications concerning things you'd like to be able to do but can't. Other people may be able to do more. But that doesn't mean you can't enjoy life as much as somebody else can. Set up reasonable goals for yourself, considering both things you have and how you feel. Then you can say that you're living your life as enjoyably as anybody else. This is more possible when you do not compare yourself with somebody else. Remember, you are you. Concentrate on making the best of your own life.

GRIEF

Grief can be an unpleasant emotion. Feelings of grief, or mourning over a loss, are common with people who have ostomies, especially right after surgery. You may grieve the loss of your intestine, your bladder, or whatever was removed. Why do you grieve? Because you're aware that you have lost something of value: in this case, a body part (as well as your bowel or urine control). Doesn't it seem strange to grieve the loss of a body part, one that is necessary for waste elimination? Remember the saying that you don't appreciate something until you lose it? And didn't you always take your excretory or urinary systems for granted? How many times did you actually say, "Thank goodness I have a working bladder/bowel?" Probably never. But now you'd like to. So you grieve the loss of this part and what it meant to you.

The loss may be either temporary or permanent. Because of it, you may feel like you have lost some physical strength. You may not like yourself as much and, subsequently, grieve this feeling of lower self-esteem.

Is grief always bad? Not necessarily. If you feel grief, then you have something very important that must be worked through. This is a very important part of the adjustment to having an ostomy.

What do you do about grief? It can't be avoided. Only by working through your grief experience will you be able to get past it and back into actual living. Crying is helpful. This doesn't mean that you should force yourself to sob. If the tears start welling up, however, don't stop yourself. Let it out. Think about what you've lost, what has changed, and what will change. Talk it out with the people you're close to. Don't ignore the fact that you have an ostomy. Otherwise, you will also be avoiding the grief process. If you want to feel better, you must work through your grief.

Mourning periods or times of grief don't last forever. You should be reassured to know that, even if you feel absolutely numb or devastated by grief, you're helping yourself by living with it. You *will* feel better!

Grief is like a deep infection. The only way to clear up certain infections is by exposing them to the air and letting them dry up. This may be painful, but eventually the wound will be completely drained and can begin to heal. See the analogy? You will reach the bottom of your grief, so that healing can begin.

UPSET

Are there times when you feel unhappy but you're not really depressed? You might feel uncomfortable but not anxious. You may not know exactly what's bothering you, or what to do about it. On the other hand, you may know exactly what's wrong, but you just don't like it. You can do things, but you'd like things to feel differently. You may feel mixed up, confused, disturbed, agitated, or shaken up. This is typical of feeling upset. Can you get upset from having an ostomy? Be serious, now!

When things happen to upset you, you may try to push them out of your mind so that you can adjust as slowly and as comfortably as possible. The stoma, appliance, and any necessary maintenance procedures are a reality, one that can't be denied or pushed away. (And if you did, think of the consequences!) So you'll have to come to grips with it.

Feeling upset is similar to experiencing other "motivating" emotions. They propel you to do something. So what should you do, now that you're all motivated? Try to figure out why you're upset. You *do* want to do something about it. There is probably something in your life that is out of sorts. Things are not moving along smoothly. Something has upset the "apple cart."

Rose was upset. A 34-year-old mother of four, she had just completed her latest car-pool adventure and was preparing to relax in front of her favorite soap opera. She had a gnawing feeling that things were just not right, and this upset her. She knew she was upset when she found that she couldn't enjoy her program. My goodness, she had been hooked on this show for almost 20 years! But she decided to turn off the t.v. and figure out what was upsetting her. After at least four commercials-worth of thought, she realized that it was her soap opera that was bothering her! She felt that the characters on the program, despite all of their script problems, were better off than she was. None of them had an ostomy—only she did! But as she thought about it, she realized that perhaps she was making something out of nothing. Actors and actresses have their own problems. So what if she also had something she must learn to live with? She *could* learn to live with an ostomy and be happy. She quickly noticed that she was feeling much better. In fact, she was able to turn on the television and breathlessly catch the last few minutes of her show!

Once you explore your upset feeling, you can act on this in much the same way as you do in attempting to resolve other emotional concerns. If you can identify the source of your upset, then plan a strategy. Otherwise, recognize that you can't, and move on.

PART III

Changes in General Lifestyle

14

Changes in General Lifestyle — An Introduction

So you have to make changes in some aspects of your lifestyle because of an ostomy? Yes, that is all part of the "package." However, changes may occur in anyone's life for a number of reasons. If you get a new job, you may have to wake up at a different time, go to work in a new direction with a new form of transportation, or "survive" on a higher salary. If your new job requires you to move, you will have to meet a whole new group of people. If there is a new addition to the family, you may have to get used to the sound of crying, changing diapers, and night feedings. In your case, there is a new addition to your life, but of a different kind: an ostomy.

Yes, there will be some changes in your lifestyle. But why assume that all of the changes have to be negative? Isn't it possible that some of them might be for the better? Maybe you were such a hard worker that you never spent enough time with your family. If you have to cut back on your work schedule because of your ostomy, maybe you'll enjoy the increased time you'll have with your family. Some of the ways you'll learn to take better care of yourself will pay off in the long run. You never know. So don't convince yourself that your life is ruined just because you have an ostomy. You should look for the positive in any situation. We'll be discussing how to deal with as many of the negatives as possible.

Following ostomy surgery, certain changes will take place. However, there are two great advantages of this surgery. First, if intestinal problems have caused chronic pain (such as inflammatory bowel disease), this pain will disappear. Second, once adjustments have taken place and you've gotten used to these changes, very few long-lasting effects will be felt.

OVERVIEW OF PART III

By reading this part of the book, you will learn how to reduce the imact of an ostomy on your lifestyle, and cope with those changes that you can't avoid. Part III includes chapters dealing with all aspects of change related to caring for your ostomy, as well as other areas of living that may be of concern, or at least of interest!

15

Taking Care
of your Ostomy

Take care of business. Ostomy business, that is. Taking care of your ostomy is an individual management concern. Whether you are managing a colostomy, an ileostomy, or a urostomy, there are as many different types of management as there are ostomates. So what do you do? Do whatever you want to and have to as long as:

1. You are comfortable.

2. Your skin remains in good condition.

3. You use appropriate appliances in economically desirable ways.

4. You control any problems you may have (such as odor or leakage).

If any of these areas give you trouble, you'll want to take steps to clear up the problem.

Management may be somewhat easier for colostomies than ileostomies because of the consistency of the stool. Colostomates have more of a working intestine. As a result, there is a better chance of water and minerals being absorbed from the food passing through. This results in a firmer residue. If the colostomy is created at the lower portion of the colon, the residue is almost completely formed into what we would normally recognize as stool. However, the higher up in the colon that elimination takes place, the looser the waste will be. Ileostomates have much less intestine remaining. This means that there is less chance of water and other materials being absorbed. Consequently, the waste is of a toothpaste-like consistency. Ileostomy management can therefore be somewhat more difficult, since there is a greater chance of leakage. As you can see, the major variables determining the specific management procedures you'll need seem to be the type of ostomy and the consistency of the waste.

How concerned are you about taking care of your ostomy? Will you have to change your lifestyle just to manage it better? Maybe you'll become so occupied with waste elimination, appliance-changing, or other management factors that you'll pay less attention to other aspects of your life. Or maybe you'll feel that the only way you can control your ostomy is by restricting your intake of fluids, figuring that this will reduce the output of fluids. This can be dangerous, so don't try to manage your ostomy this way.

Is this concern so necessary? Not on your life. You may have to make some changes, but you certainly shouldn't become a different person. Learn to efficiently manage your ostomy and you'll cope better with "taking care of business."

FITTING APPLIANCES

Wearing an appliance involves more than just slapping a pouch against your abdomen and letting it do its thing! A proper fit is essential for efficiency as well as comfort. At first, right after surgery, you probably won't be able to fit yourself with your appliance. You probably won't even know how to select appliances, but you'll learn! You'll receive instructions on preparing the skin, applying any skin barrier, applying the adhesive, putting on the appliance, and making sure that the appliance fits properly. It won't be long before you're an expert in taking care of your ostomy needs. You may be saying, "Wonderful. Just what I need, to be an ostomy expert." But think about it. The faster you really know what you're doing, the sooner your ostomy will become a routine part of you.

When fitting the appliances, it's very important to attach the adhesive or face plate properly. The face plate should be just a little bit larger than the opening of the stoma. If it is too large, waste material may touch your skin between the opening of the face plate and the stoma, causing irritation. Leakage could also be a problem if the face plate is too large. If you have a urostomy, it is recommended that the space between the face plate or appliance and the opening of the stoma be no more than one sixteenth of an inch. If you're a colostomate or an ileostomate, about an eighth of an inch should be permitted. This allows for expansion of the stoma itself.

Fitting appliances require a little more care in children. Why? As children grow, the shape and even the location of the stoma may change. As a result, you'll want to make sure that appliances continue to fit properly. Otherwise, leakage or skin irritation can be frequent problems. Every ostomate, child through adult, needs to have appliances that fit properly, prevent leakage and odor, and maximize feelings of security and comfort.

CHANGING APPLIANCES

Changing your appliance is a basic part of ostomy management. It refers to the act of removing the appliance and replacing it with a new one. This is not to be confused with emptying the appliance, which we'll discuss in the next section.

Is this hard to do? Not at all. You'll easily learn the procedures necessary for changing appliances. It just takes practice. As a matter of fact, changing two-piece systems can be as easy as snapping or unsnapping Tupperware! Obviously, younger children may have a harder time, and the very young will not be able to do it at all. Therefore, parents should be present immediately following surgery, to learn the proper methods for changing appliances. They will then be able to teach the child as he or she becomes old enough to handle it alone.

How often should you change appliances? Usually, pouches can be used from five to seven days before discarding, as long as they are emptied regularly, cleansed properly, and the skin surrounding the stoma is well protected. Some people even try to wear them longer. But if you do, be careful!

You may find that, in hot or humid weather, appliances have to be changed more often. Adhesives may not hold up as well at such times. If you sweat, the appliance may not adhere to your skin as well. It may have to be changed more often, not necessarily because it is full, but to avoid leakage resulting from an inadequate fit.

Because urine is a liquid, there are differences between changing urostomy appliances and ileostomy or colostomy appliances. If you have a urostomy, you particularly want to try to change at a time when your ostomy is less active. You may find that, like many urostomates, once the initial flow of urine in the morning is over, activity is usually quiet enough to facilitate changing. Do this before doing any more drinking. Ileostomates usually find it best to change appliances either right before meals or several hours after meals. Ostomies tend to be more active within one or two hours after you eat.

EMPTYING AND DISPOSING APPLIANCES

Your pouch has enough in it, and it's time to empty. Now what do you do? What's the best way to dispose of the contents or the whole appliance? This may start off as a long, unpleasant procedure, especially if you are a new ostomate. It'll become more tolerable as you turn "pro." But nobody is thrilled to touch his or her excretions. In fact, contact with waste is something that has always been discouraged. You've probably avoided it since you were little. But now you don't have a choice. You'll be more in contact with waste matter, feces and urine, than you ever were or ever wanted to be. To minimize any unpleasantness, you'll want to learn efficiency. Efficiency leads to emptying appliances quickly and with little difficulty.

The type of appliance will help determine the actual disposal procedure. In some cases, appliances will just be discarded. In other cases, they will be emptied and washed out or simply drained. With one-piece, open-ended, drainable systems, whether disposable or permanent, you can usually flush out the pouch from the bottom and then close the end. One-piece, closed-end systems are simply removed and replaced. With two-piece systems, the pouch can simply be detached from the face plate, and either cleansed and reapplied or discarded.

Ileostomy appliances, as well as urostomy appliances, are usually emptied directly into the toilet. The drainage of the urostomy appliance is almost similar to urinating. The emptying of an ileostomy appliance, however, may cause splattering if held too high above the bowl when emptied. Even if it is lowered, some splattering may occur, something you certainly don't want! Try flushing the toilet at the moment of emptying. This will reduce the chances of splattering.

Deciding how often you should empty your appliance is an individual choice. First of all, it depends on the type of ostomy you have. For example, if you have an end colostomy, you may be able to wear the appliance longer before emptying it. This is because you're better able to tell when the appliance is filling up. If you are an ileostomate, you'll also get to know how long you can put off emptying. But because there is less firmness in the feces, you'll have to be more aware of the capacity of the appliance and when it should be emptied. This is necessary to avoid spillage or other problems. If you're a urostomate, your appliance must be monitored most carefully. When your appliance becomes too full of urine, the chances of leakage increase significantly.

Decisions involving when to empty the appliance also depend on your activities. If you're about to participate in strenuous exercise, for example, you may want to empty immediately before starting. The same applies to the start of a prolonged trip, regardless of the type of transportation. You may prefer to empty your appliance before you go to sleep. Or you might prefer to empty your appliance in the morning after you awaken. If you do not want to empty your appliance at night, try to alter your eating schedule so that you eat major meals earlier in the day. Given time, you'll learn what your preferences are, based on experience and trial-and-error.

You may find it better to schedule drainage times, rather than simply waiting until the appliance is full. Set up a regular routine for yourself. Do this as soon as you're aware of the appliance that is best for you and how your body works in eliminating waste. This will provide the most reassuring atmosphere and the most security against leakage. In addition, you'll always know when to put aside time for this activity and where you're going to do it. Obviously, your schedule is not carved in stone. But you'll have a better idea of how to organize your day. Appliance maintenance will become a part of your regular routine. This helps in the adjustment process because it is a "part of you."

SPECIAL UROSTOMY CONSIDERATIONS

Urostomy appliances should be drained frequently to prevent urine from coming in contact with the skin around the stoma. Even drops of urine coming in contact with the skin can potentially cause irritation. You'll learn what "frequently" means for you. This depends on stoma placement, the extent your stoma protrudes, and your body condition, as well as your output, the size of your appliance, your activity, and your age, among other factors.

No More Wet Dreams

Take special precautions at night. You might want to use a special night drainage appliance. This is actually a second appliance, which collects urine from the primary appliance. It may be as simple as a plastic jug or bottle. Using it lessens the chance of your main appliance overflowing and, as a result, it is less likely for your sleep to be interrupted. Your appliance will remain more securely attached to your abdomen if urine doesn't quickly fill it up. Another reason to use a second drainage appliance is so that urine will not collect in one place for a long time. This can be a breeding ground for bacteria that can cause very serious infections. So make sure you collect urine in appliances that will keep it as far away from the skin and stoma as possible. The night drainage appliance may be located on the side of the bed so that tubing from the primary appliance drains urine directly into this other collection device.

Using an extra drainage bottle may also be helpful if you are going on a long trip, or if there is any other reason why you might want to empty your appliance less often. In these situations, you may want to use a leg appliance. This is actually an added urine collecting device, which you attach to the lower part of your leg. Because more urine can collect before you empty, you won't have to empty as frequently.

DISCARDING

In general, it's better to throw away empty appliances. This makes sense with urostomates and ileostomates. However, some colostomates feel the urge to take the whole appliance, contents and all, and throw it away. This, if done carefully, is sometimes feasible. If not, you may want to open the appliance, either through the top or by using an old pair of scissors or a knife to cut it open. Flush away the contents and then discard the appliance.

WHAT ABOUT CHILDREN?

It's usually necessary for children to empty or change their appliances more frequently than adults. Why? Children are usually more active and not as skilled in managing the ostomy. Also, children are frequently not as careful in protecting themselves. They may not be as careful in the actual emptying or changing process. Because of this, it may be necessary for adult supervision to continue, as well as for added cleanliness to be practiced during and following the change. Another reason why children may have to empty or change appliances more often is because of their size. Because they are smaller, they must wear smaller appliances. Smaller appliances will hold less, and therefore have to be emptied and changed more often.

CLEANING APPLIANCES

When emptying or changing appliances, they should be thoroughly cleaned. If disposables are used, this is not as much of a problem, since you may get rid of them anyway. But if permanent appliances are used, they must be thoroughly cleaned following emptying. The cleaning of appliances is necessary to eliminate odor. In addition, clean appliances last longer, are less likely to cause skin irritations around the stoma, and are less likely to leak. If cleaning does not eliminate residue, any mineral salts, or other problems (such as odor), the appliance should be discarded. Rubber appliances, for example, may be less effective in repelling odors after being used for six months or more.

How do you clean your appliances? You can scrub them or soak them (usually 30 minutes is sufficient) in antiseptic-type solutions. These solutions are usually suggested by the manufacturers of the product, since they're the ones who should know what's best for each appliance! In addition, you can use other preparations that have been designed for appliance cleaning. If you wash them, you're probably better off using lukewarm or cool water, but never hot water. Hot water opens up the pores of the appliances (like it does to your skin) and increases the chance of absorbing odor.

Following any cleaning procedure, rinse thoroughly and allow appliances to dry completely. You'll probably want to rotate appliances, using one while another one that has just been cleaned is drying out. This is better than using the same one.

YOUR SKIN

Clean skin is usually healthy skin. If your skin is smooth and cared for, your appliance will fit better and more comfortably. You'll even be able to wear it longer. On the other hand, if your skin is not clean, irritation may result. This can affect the fit of the appliance. If it doesn't fit securely, additional problems may result (can you guess which ones?).

Another important reason for your skin to be carefully maintained is because of the excessive "wear and tear." You'll frequently have to remove and replace appliances. So you'll want to be gentle and diligent in keeping your skin clean.

Any time you change your appliance, the skin should be cleaned very carefully. The skin should be washed with non-detergent soap and water. Make sure that all soap is removed when you are finished. If you want to make sure that the stoma is clean and well taken care of, use very soft tissues or light gauze to gently damp or blot it. Be gentle! Even wiping can create an irritation or cause bleeding. It is not unusual for a tiny blood vessel (a capillary) to "pop" and dribble a little blood. This is normal, so don't panic! This bleeding will usually stop when washing is complete. Stomas should be kept clean and irritation-free. You also want to protect your stoma from injury.

Once your skin is completely clean, you're still not finished. You'll want to apply a skin barrier. If your skin is healthy and intact, this may be all you need. For added protection, you may want to use a gel, adhesive, or karaya. If you notice any signs of skin irritation, applications should include skin treatments to help soothe the irritation.

How About Bathing?

Will bathing routines be the same as before? Can showers or baths be taken with freedom? Should you wear your appliance? This all depends on the type of ostomy you have. In general, showers and baths are completely safe. The problem is the concern about waste discharge. People with sigmoid or descending colostomies, for example, may sit in a bathtub without appliances. This is usually not the case if you have an ileostomy or urostomy. You don't want the unpleasantness of waste being discharged during a bath, contaminating the water. If you have a "draining" ostomy, you're probably better off wearing your pouch and taking a shower instead of a bath. You can shower without the appliance, of course, if you're not concerned about a discharge from the stoma. But for baths, bandages over the stoma probably wouldn't help. Wearing your appliance in the tub is not usually recommended, since the seal may soften and weaken. But what about the stoma? Stomas need not be washed (except during appliance-changing, to remove any fecal matter that remains). They don't even require as much care as the skin. There is nothing wrong, however, with allowing them to be uncovered during a bath or shower.

Is Bathing Safe?

Bathing is nearly always safe for ostomates. Bath water cannot return to the body through a stoma. This is because of peristalsis, the motion that keeps waste material moving in an outward direction. In addition, one-way valves prevent this in some ostomies. However, in pyelostomies and nephrostomies (two types of urostomies), water may return through the openings and cause problems. It can back up into the bladder or kidneys, increasing the chance of infection. So if you have this type of ostomy and want to take a bath, make sure that the water level remains below the level of your stoma.

Irritation

You may find this section irritating! Why? Regardless of how much you try to prevent skin irritation (also called excoriation), it may be unavoidable from time to time. Proper care reduces your chances of skin irritation. However, let's talk about what happens when skin does become irritated and what you can do about it.

Irritated skin may simply start out being tender, then sore, with a more reddish color than usual. It may become encrusted or inflamed, broken or cracked. This can be quite painful and you probably wouldn't want anything to touch your skin during this time. But you'll have to, because of both the need for skin treatments and the fact that you need to wear your appliances (and clothes, for that matter!). Unfortunately, you may need to change your appliance more frequently because of your skin's condition. Irritation can affect the fitting of the appliance. The fitting may have to be temporarily readjusted.

What May Cause Irritations?

What cleaning agents are you using on your skin? It's possible that they are causing reactions. Does your skin have any particular reaction to adhesives you may use? Are you letting waste material accumulate on the skin? This may happen because your appliance is not being changed frequently enough, because of leakage, or because of overflow.

What to Do

Pay attention to your skin's condition. Watch for any signs of irritation, pimples, spots, or breaks in the skin. If you see any signs of problems with the skin, attend to them immediately. Try to improve your skin condition by using lotions, creams, or other simple treatment methods. If your skin becomes raw or sore, or there are signs of infections, bring this to the attention of a professional right away.

There are treatment powders or adhesives that can be used. These may be somewhat different from those that you use regularly. If you have a continent ileostomy or control your stoma using irrigation, the dressing itself (which is applied to the stoma) can contain medication or treatment. Some ostomates have found that applying soothing oils, such as Vitamin E oil, can be very helpful. The problem with this, however, is the difficulty of affixing an appliance to oily skin.

STOMA STABILITY

Remember the song, *No Matter What Shape Your Stomach Is In?* It was the theme song of a popular Alka-Seltzer commercial. But we're changing it. Now we'll call it, *It Matters What Shape Your Stoma Is In!* You should examine your stoma on a regular basis. What should you look for? First, make sure that your stoma remains approximately the same size (after healing is complete, usually after six months). If the size of your stoma changes significantly, bring this to the attention of your physician. How does your stoma look? Do you see any changes in appearance? Has the color changed at all? Has its texture changed? If you see any changes in color or shape, or if you see new little spots, bring this to a professional's attention. A healthy stoma will serve you well. A damaged stoma will cause you problems. Keep on top of things (and that doesn't mean resting on your abdomen all day!).

PERINEAL PROBLEMS

Did you have your rectum and anus removed as part of your ostomy surgery? If so, you have what is called a perineal wound. The gap left in the perineum when the rectum and anus are removed requires a great deal of care.

The perineal area can be quite tender and sore for a long time. You may feel like you'll never be able to sit comfortably again. Eating and watching t.v. standing up is no fun! The area may take a long time to heal, because it takes a long time for scar tissue to fill the opening. How long? The amount of time varies from person to person. You may find that the wound has healed completely in less than two months. Sometimes it may take more than a year. That's quite a range. What factors contribute to this range? Consider the following questions. How extensive was the surgery? What kind of operation was it? How big was the wound itself? What was your surgeon's choice of procedure for closing the wound? Are you eating properly? How active are you? Aren't these exciting questions? Hold on, there's more! What was your physical condition before surgery? Did you have any pre-existing scar tissue in the area? What shape is your pelvis (no photographs, please)? Have you been using any medication, such as steroids (which may slow down healing)? Enough already. The answers may have a bearing on how long it takes for perineal wounds to heal.

Another problem is that the perineal area does not usually have such a good flow of blood. Good blood circulation is very important in promoting healing. It is important that the outer part of the skin does not heal before the inner part. If this occurs, abscesses or fistulae may form. Fluid may accumulate in these areas, forming pockets, and infection can set in. What do surgeons do to try to prevent this from happening? Some surgeons pack the wound with gauze and leave it open. This allows it to heal from the inside out, with the opening getting smaller and smaller. Other surgeons believe that the skin should be stitched together. This requires drainage tubes, so that blood or other fluids can drain out of the area. Absorbent pads may be used to absorb this discharge. As healing takes place, the amount of discharge decreases.

So What Can You Do?

While you're waiting for the perineal area to heal, you'll be more comfortable sitting on a soft cushion. But it's usually not a good idea to sit on a "doughnut," or any cushion with a hole cut in the middle. This might cause the skin to stretch outward, put more of a strain on the perineal area, and produce pain! Stretching the area can also slow down healing.

Sitz baths can be very soothing and helpful. Park your derriere in warm, circulating water. Not only is this pleasant, relaxing, and comfortable, but it can stimulate better blood circulation. This promotes healing.

To reduce the healing time for perineal wounds, keep the area clean! Avoiding infection is a must! In addition to washing the area using sitz baths or direct cleaning, another procedure that is occasionally used is called "lamping". A special lamp (you can even use a regular incandescent lamp) is placed where the heat generated from the light can help dry the area completely. There is very little irritation, since no skin is touched.

Finally, Beware of the "Phantom"

Did you ever hear of the "phantom limb" phenomenon? That's when someone has had a limb amputated, but feels as though it's still there. You may even have an occasional desire to look and see if it is there. This phenomenon also occurs when the rectum has been removed. "Phantom" rectal feelings can give you the feeling of a full bowel, along with the need to defecate. Sound strange? Be assured that this feeling is not unusual. It comes from the triggering of nerves in the spinal cord. It doesn't mean that any part of the perineum has been left intact. Phantom sensations will decrease in time. But if you're uncomfortable, sometimes just sitting on the toilet for a short period of time can help. This will reassure you that the feeling is a phantom one.

16

Irrigation

"Wait, I've heard that term before. Doesn't it refer to the process by which farmers improve their crops?" No, Zeke, this is a book on coping with ostomies, not coping with dry spells! For colostomates, irrigation is a regulating procedure. You use it to try and regain some control over the times when waste is expelled. Water enters the intestine through the stoma. (This doesn't happen by accident, by the way. You squirt it in). The water causes the bowel to expand or distend. (It is not used to wash out the colon.) After this, when the bowel contracts, the presence of the water triggers peristaltic movement, which forces out the waste material. Irrigation is similar to enema procedures, but it is done through the stoma. It is usually not done on temporary colostomies, but is primarily used with permanent ones.

Irrigation procedures are the most popular among individuals with sigmoid colostomies. It is a popular method of management used in the United States.

Many colostomates like the feeling of control. It is almost like "the way it used to be" before colostomy surgery. Another reason for its popularity is because it decreases the costs involved in colostomy care. You'll save money that would otherwise be spent on appliances, and irrigation equipment usually lasts a long time. It is not nearly as popular in other countries. One reason for this is the cost factor. In many other countries, appliances used for colostomy management are free. So saving money would not be an incentive to using irrigation, as it might be in the U.S. Another possibility? In other countries, families are more likely to have only one bathroom. Nobody likes a tied-up bathroom, and irrigation does take time. Family members who aren't irrigating may object to being shut out.

MUST YOU IRRIGATE?

If you irrigate, you're one of thousands of colostomates who do this to try to improve the ability to control or regulate the elimination of waste. There are many others, however, who want little to do with the process, and won't irrigate. In general, older ostomates are less likely to irrigate than younger ostomates.

Must you irrigate? No. Are you afraid that, without irrigation, your intestines may become impacted or infected or result in other complications? Not true. Before your colostomy, did you use an enema to regulate your bowels? So why feel that you need irrigation now? If you were to use it, you'd only be using it voluntarily to try to retain some control over the waste flow.

Irrigation can be helpful from time to time, even if you don't use it regularly. On those infrequent occasions when impaction does occur, or constipation cannot be relieved, you may want to irrigate.

HOW DOES IT WORK?

How does the irrigating process work? Irrigation actually "teaches" the still-functioning segment of the colon how to "behave." The colon learns how to respond to the water flow by eliminating waste. If the colon is a good student and learns properly, the bowel will not eliminate waste when water is not introduced. The waste material accumulates in the colon until the water starts the irrigation response (not to be confused with the relaxation response!). If it works, you're in control. You can regulate the elimination of waste. Until water comes inside the bowel, you really don't have to worry about the expulsion of waste.

DOES IT ALWAYS WORK?

If you do regulate by irrigation, will you always be "successful?" Not always. You may not be able to regulate your bowel using irrigation even if you wanted to. Some bowels simply do not respond to regulating procedures. The types of food you eat may have a bearing on how well irrigation works. Some foods (such as low-residue foods) may not "bulk" as well, decreasing your chances for irrigation success.

Another sign that irrigation is not working is if you don't flush out all accumulated waste. Incomplete elimination may be due to more than just the types of food you eat. One reason may be constipation. Even a flow of water cannot sufficiently loosen very firm waste material so it can be discharged. Excessive fatigue, dehydration, stress, or emotional strain may all contribute to irrigation problems. Being in a hurry may also result in an incomplete irrigation. Do you take tranquilizers? This, too, can have its effect. The tranquilizer may slow down the movement of the colon as it slows down the rest of the body.

WHEN TO BEGIN?

By now you've read all about why colostomates irrigate, what it does, when it may not work, and other assorted goodies. Have you decided to try it? First make sure that your physician gives you the green light.

Usually, you won't begin irrigation procedures until a number of weeks after surgery. This is because it's harder to regulate discharge right away, since there can be a more continuous flow of waste during the time following surgery. You'll wear appliances during this interval, but you can still gear up for the beginning of irrigation. How? Start observing elimination activity. Notice any consistent time patterns that will be helpful when you want to start irrigating. Your physician will let you know when the time is appropriate to begin colonic irrigations.

WHAT DO YOU DO?

You'll usually sit on the toilet (or a chair next to the toilet) after filling an irrigation bag with about a quart of lukewarm water. This irrigation bag is suspended at approximately shoulder-height, or even a little bit higher, so that gravity draws the water through a tube into the stoma. The tube is carefully inserted through the stoma and has a plastic cone lubricated for comfortable placement. The cone usually fits snugly, preventing any possibility of intestinal damage. (This occurred occasionally with previous methods of irrigation, such as using a catheter.) Irrigation kits usually contain special appliances (irrigation sleeves) that attach around the stoma. There are openings at the top, so that the tube from the suspended bag goes right through it and into the stoma. There is an opening at the bottom, from which the discharge flows into the toilet. What about the tube? For your convenience it usually contains a valve that lets you regulate the speed of the water flow into the stoma. If it does not contain a valve, you can always pinch the tubing to regulate the flow. With experience, you'll learn the proper pressure of water that is best for you.

It usually takes approximately eight to ten minutes for the quart of water to flow into the intestine. You'll then wait another five minutes or so before removing the cone and tube, or catheter. At that time, waste will begin to flow out of the stoma, usually in spurts. The spurts go through the irrigation sleeve and drop into the toilet. This discharge phase of the irrigation procedure can take forty-five minutes or more. Does that mean you have to sit and wait for the whole time? No. After the first ten to twenty minutes, most of the waste has been eliminated. At this point, you may want to fold over the bottom of the irrigation sleeve, clip it securely, and proceed with other activities while the rest of the process is completed. It won't take too long for you to learn how you'll feel at each stage of the process. As you gain confidence in this process, you will be less fearful of accidents between irrigations. You may not even feel the need to wear appliances. You might just want to use a pad of some type to protect the stoma. Not only will this pad protect the stoma, but it will also guard against any possible mucous discharge or slight waste discharge. Your irrigation kit may come with special pouches that can be applied over the stoma after irrigation.

HOW OFTEN SHOULD YOU IRRIGATE?

Successful irrigation to completely flush out the waste is rarely needed more than every 24 hours. In order to regulate bowel movements, you may want to irrigate at the same time every day (preferably after a meal, since this stimulates peristalsis). If you find that bowel movements are still not occurring daily, you may decide to irrigate every other day or, in some cases, every third or fourth day. You'll learn by experimenting.

A FINAL INSERTION

Irrigation is not for every colostomate. It's up to you to decide whether or not you want to try it. If you do decide to irrigate, it can be very helpful. Remember: after every successful irrigation, you'll probably feel flushed with victory!

17

Ostomy Management Concerns

In addition to the "normal" parts of caring for your ostomy, there are some things that you probably worry about, right? I don't know any ostomate who hasn't, at one time or another, worried about leakage, odor, or gas. So let's discuss these three anticipated "day-ruiners" and see what can be done to put your mind (and body) at ease.

LEAKAGE

Have you ever been apprehensive about leakage or is this the understatement of the year? One of the primary concerns of every ostomate is leakage. Fear of "telltale spots" appearing on clothing, puddles, or other signs, can be very anxiety-provoking.

If leakage does occur, why did it happen? Because the appliance had a tiny hole in it? Because it was not securely fastened to the skin surrounding your stoma? Because your appliance overflowed or was too full? What other reasons might there be? Checking carefully decreases the chances of it happening again. Is your skin irritated? If so, this can affect the way the appliance fits, increasing the chances of an unpleasant event. So always take preventive measures.

Leakage is more likely to occur in an ileostomate or transverse colostomate than an end colostomate. Since the latter's waste material is more firm, it is less likely to leak. Softer waste in the former may lead to a greater chance of leakage. Obviously, therefore, which ostomates have the greatest chance of leakage? You guessed it—the urostomates.

As it fills up, the appliance becomes heavier. You may be concerned that it will put more of a strain on the adhesive or face plate. Wearing a belt can provide more support for the appliance, but this doesn't necessarily eliminate the chance of leakage. Belts are not worn as frequently these days because adhesives are improving in quality and reliability. On the other hand, children are more likely to wear belts. Why? They may not be as careful in taking proper care of their appliances or emptying them frequently enough. The belt will provide some extra protection.

Avoiding embarrassment is not the only reason to try to prevent leakage. Spilled waste can be a problem for the skin. If digestive enzymes are still contained in the stool, these may cause an irritation.

So how do you protect against leakage? Be sure of a proper appliance fit, clean and change it when appropriate, and inspect it frequently to make sure that there are no defects. Use proper appliances and proper adhesives. Make sure there is a secure seal and fit around the stoma. These are the best ways to protect against leakage.

ODOR

Are you afraid of odor? (Unpleasant odor, of course!) Odor is one of the biggest concerns of ostomates. There are two types of odor: odor from the waste material itself and odor from gas. (More on gas later in this chapter). Urostomates are usually not as concerned with odor as ileostomates or colostomates. This is because properly-diluted urine rarely has a foul odor.

Every individual, whether an ostomate or not, has odor in his stool. It cannot be avoided. The intensity of the odor varies from person to person, from time to time, from situation to situation. It is as unique as your fingerprint (but it *won't* be recorded by the F.B.I.!). Although odor is not totally preventable, it can be dealt with. How? We'll get to that. (But as a "sneak preview," either modifications in diet or the use of artificial additives can be helpful.)

Odor-provokers

What causes odor? The types of food you eat may have something to do with it. Certain foods are more likely than others to create odor. Foods such as onions, garlic, or different types of shellfish, can produce odor.

But what you eat isn't the only culprit. Certain medications or infections may cause odors. After a period of time, odor may be given off from the appliance itself, especially those that are made of rubber.

Odor-Busters

How can you control odor? By taking better care of the very things that cause odor: diet and your appliance. Diet control may include eating parsley (a great natural deodorizer) or avoiding foods that cause gas or odor (such as asparagus—a problem for urostomates). Drink plenty of fluids, especially cranberry juice. This is a great way to reduce any foul odor in the urine. It works by maintaining a proper level of acidity. The extra fluids dilute the urine. More on this in the chapter, *Weight Changes and Nutritional Needs*.

Cleaning appliances is another important way to prevent odor. Clean appliances do not smell. Many good preparations are useful in deodorizing your appliance. Hydrogen peroxide, for example, may be helpful. Any of the inexpensive or commercial mouthwashes available can help. Even breath mints, sprays, or drops can be used if nothing else is available. One thing that should never be used, however, is aspirin. Although aspirin can neutralize odor, it could cause severe irritations or skin ulcers if it comes in contact with the stoma or the lining of the intestine. In addition to aspirin, no preparations containing alcohol should be used, since these can also irritate the skin. But don't go crazy and spend lots of money on preparations, deodorants, detergents, and the like. You don't want to produce results that are even worse than the very odors you're trying to eliminate!

The Cleanliness Factor

There are two other very important things to keep in mind when minimizing odor. The first is cleanliness. Although that may seem obvious, it's worth repeating. It is important to be as clean as possible in order to prevent odors.

The second rule is that the appliance used should be one that does not absorb odor. For this reason, it's not a good idea to use rubber appliances for more than six months. In addition, you're probably better off washing your appliance in cool or cold water. (As I mentioned earlier, hot water opens the pores of the appliance, allowing odors to be absorbed by the appliance material). Your appliance should also be odor-proof, one that confines odors inside and prevents them from escaping or leaking. If gas is a cause of odor and your appliance is used with a gas-release valve, these valves should have built-in deodorizers. In this way, the gas that is released is deodorized as it escapes.

If you are searching for appliances that will do the best job for you, keep in mind that there is a difference between those advertised as *odor-proof* and those that are *odor-resistant*. *Odor-proof* appliances are considered to be 100% effective in controlling odor. *Odor-resistant* ones, although effective, may not be infallible.

An Olfactory Overview

If the natural techniques we've discussed so far are not working, and artificial preparations, (either in mouth or in pouch) are not successful, a physician should be consulted. No medications or preparations should be taken without a physician's approval. Any preparations that are being used in the pouch should be checked for ingredients. Make sure they will not be harmful to the skin. If you're in doubt as to what can be used to clean the skin or put in the appliance, just remember: if you can put it in your mouth, you can use it around your stoma. With proper attention, odor can be controlled.

GAS

Are you concerned about a "gas explosion" when you are with people? Most ostomates are. Of course, it's not nearly the same problem when you're alone, but even so . . . ! There are two problems with gas (or flatus, as it's medically called): the noise (it's not music to anyone's ears) and the smell (which can be even more embarrassing). Why can gas be a problem for ostomates? The newly-created stoma has no sphincter. Non-ostomates have anal sphincter muscles, which help to control the passage of gas. Because the stoma does not contain these muscles, the passage of gas cannot be controlled. Gas can make noise. Because it comes from an opening on the abdomen rather than between the legs, it can be more noticeable. This is because gas escaping between the legs is muffled by layers of skin, as well as layers of clothing. For ostomates, only the clothing is able to muffle the sound.

What causes gas? Some foods contributing to the passage of gas are those in the cucumber family or lentil family (such as dried beans). Chewing gum can also cause gas problems, since air may be swallowed along with the saliva. Carbonated beverages can be troublesome as well. Gas can come from the release of swallowed air. It results from bacterial action as well as other chemical reactions that normally occur in the intestines.

Ostomates usually notice the most gas immediately following surgery. This is because the intestines take time to settle down and resume normal activity. Problems may arise if the gas passes into the appliance. The pouch may swell from the increased pressure inside. Some ostomates feel like puncturing the appliance to allow the gas to escape. This isn't a good idea, unless you're in a position to reseal the puncture. If so, use a patch that will not allow odor or matter to escape.

Causing a Gas Shortage

Some appliances have safety valves that are used primarily to release the excessive build-up of gas. If this is the case, make sure that the safety valve has a special closure so that it's easily controllable. Charcoal filters in this valve may be quite desirable, so that the unpleasant odor can be filtered out of the gas as it escapes.

What you put in your mouth can also help you to control the gas problem. Antacids and certain foods (such as yogurt) can help to control gas. The way you chew is very important. Regardless of what you eat, chew foods carefully for longer periods of time and be careful not to swallow air along with the food. In order to reduce the amount of air swallowed while eating, try to chew with your mouth closed. Do you chew with your mouth open? If you do, you'll be breathing by mouth while chewing and swallowing. You'll swallow much more air than you'd like to.

Eating regular meals can also help, since avoiding food can cause gas. Sometimes, it's a good idea to have six small meals a day instead of three regular meals. In this way, the stomach always has something in it and the digestive processes always have something to work on.

18

Problems or Complications

Ostomy surgery is not the most pleasant experience. But at least you hope that it will take care of the problems necessitating it. You also hope that there will be no recurrence of the problem (please!). Actually, you probably hope that you'll never need surgery again!

PROBLEMS

No ostomate has ever been completely problem-free. But you can cope more successfully with your ostomy if you're aware of possible problems and have some idea what to do about them.

Bleeding

Slight bleeding, if it does occur, is not necessarily a reason for alarm. However, it should be observed very closely, especially if you notice a foul odor or any signs of pus. Because the stoma is so sensitive, stomal bleeding is not unusual. If it continues for a prolonged period of time, however, let your physician know. Also, notify your physician if you notice any blood in the stool or, for that matter, any significant changes in the stool. This may indicate problems in the remaining intestinal tract.

Infection

Any signs of infection should also be reported to your physician. Anyone can get an infection and you, as an ostomate, are no exception. If you're a urostomate, you may be particularly prone to infections because of the change in the way urine flows out of the body. We've mentioned before that urine should not be able to flow back either into the stoma or the kidneys themselves. Do you remember why? If urine accumulates either in the kidneys or in the tubes leading out of the body, bacteria may grow very rapidly, greatly increasing your susceptibility to infection. One way to avoid kidney infections is to drink plenty of water. This keeps the kidneys flushed and the urine diluted. If the urine does not become too concentrated or alkaline, there is less chance of infection from bacterial growth. Drinking cranberry juice or taking Vitamin C tablets can also keep the urine from being too alkaline. Cleaning appliances is very important for urostomates, probably more than for anyone else. Thorough cleaning also reduces the possibilities of infection.

Ileostomates and colostomates are also susceptible to infections. They may develop within the intestine itself or in the stoma and are usually noticed if a foul odor (different from the one you are used to) fills your nostrils. You may also notice an infection if pus is discharged from the area. Physicians should be immediately informed of any signs of infection so that treatment can begin.

Constipation

Constipation may be another problem requiring special management. Very hard stool may be difficult to pass through the stoma. Commercial stool softeners may be helpful, although in some cases they may be more trouble than they're worth. Try eating foods containing more bulk or residue, such as bran, fruits and vegetables, or breads made from whole grain. This may be helpful in moving things along! Drinking lots of fluids, including a little morning prune juice, can also help. Other suggestions for alleviating constipation include warm baths, drinking cups of hot liquid, and exercising. Although these activities do not directly affect the feces, they may promote better peristaltic movement and smoother intestinal passage.

Obstructions

Obstructions or blockages may be a problem for ileostomates and colostomates. Certain foods, such as nuts or popcorn, may affect the feces themselves. If you don't chew your food properly or if you swallow large pieces, this may also cause you to become clogged. When ileostomy blockages occur, it may be helpful to gently irrigate the area. However, this should never be done without a physician's approval.

If you are a colostomate or ileostomate, the best way to prevent blockages is to observe some basic nutritional and digestive rules. For example, drink proper amounts of fluids and eat a well-balanced diet containing proper amounts of roughage. Get enough exercise to maintain good physical tone. Gently massage your abdomen, bring your knees up to your chest, or take a warm bath. This might help. Finally, remember that your emotions can have a bearing on blockages and obstructions. Learn how to cope with your emotions as much as possible. (Reread Part II at least eighteen times!)

If, after all these suggestions, you're still having difficulty, maybe the blockage is related to physical problems, such as stricture (reduced size) in the intestine or a narrowing of the stoma opening. Other problems causing blockage might be a sharp bend in the intestine, internal swelling, irritation, or herniation either in the intestine or near the stoma. These and other such problems, although troublesome, can usually be resolved by surgery, if other attempts don't work.

COMPLICATIONS

Unfortunately, complications do occur occasionally, although perhaps even less frequently than the problems described above. It's important that you be aware of this, although this doesn't mean that you should become obsessed with the possibilities. The type of complication we're discussing depends on the type of ostomy surgery you've had. Among the potential complications that may occur following ostomy surgery are: hernias, abcesses, fistulae, kidney stones, stricturing, prolapse, retraction, stenosis, excoriation, or injury. Whew! One at a time, please!

Hernias

Hernias may occur in the area near your stoma. Or, in some cases, they may occur at the very site of the stoma. Why? When an opening is created in the abdominal wall (as in the opening for your stoma), the surgery may cut muscles that are used to maintain firmness and abdominal strength. The resulting weakness may allow part of the intestine to sneak through the abdominal wall! Although most careful surgery minimizes the chances of these hernias, you can help too! Avoid heavy lifting or other strenuous exercise, which may put added strain on already weakened abdominal muscles.

Abcesses or Fistulae

Following the removal of the rectum, fistulae or abcesses may occur in the perineal area if the outer layers of skin close before the inner layers do. Pockets may form, in which fluid can accumulate and become infected. Taking good care of this area following surgery reduces the incidence of the problem. Abcesses or fistulae may occur in other places in the intestinal tract as well.

Kidney Stones

Kidney stones are another potential complication following ostomy surgery. If you have either an ileostomy or urostomy, you have a greater chance of developing kidney stones than if you had other surgery. But this doesn't mean it'll happen to you. If complications do occur, kidney stones are one of the more common types. Fortunately, some kidney stones pass normally and do not require surgery. However, if they last for awhile and cause a lot of discomfort (and other efforts to eliminate them have not been successful), surgery may be necessary. What's the best way to avoid kidney stones? Remember that dehydration is one of the most common causes of kidney stones. So drink plenty of fluids. This will continually flush out your kidneys, reducing the build-up of stone-forming matter.

Stricturing

Stricture, or narrowing, is a problem that occurs more with urostomates than with any other type of ostomate. Why? The waste passageway in ileostomies or colostomies is usually wider than the tubes used in urostomies. Urostomy tubes (ureters) are narrow to begin with. Further narrowing of the ureters can be dangerous, since this would make it harder for the urine to flow and a backup might cause problems. Stricturing may be caused by an accumulation of matter (possibly because of urine that is too alkaline) on the walls of the tubes.

Other Complications

Problems with the stoma itself, such as prolapse (where more of the intestine comes out) or retraction (where the stoma pulls in), may also occur. Stomal stenosis is a type of scarring that usually results from prolonged inflammation. Occasionally, stenosis occurs in the ileal segment of an ileal conduit. Stomal stenosis may also occur if the stoma does not protrude far enough away from the skin. This can occur in any type of ostomy. Keeping the urine acidic (rather than alkaline) can help to reduce the inflammation that may result in urostomy scarring (and, as mentioned above, will also help avoid stricturing problems). Once scarring occurs it may be irreversible. In this case, scarring can only be treated through further surgery.

Another complication related to stomal stenosis is excoriation of the skin. This, or other intense skin irritation, can come as a result of many different things. Primarily, however, it occurs when there is too much contact between the skin and waste material. Usually, the contact occurs around the stoma and under the appliance face plate. Once skin excoriation occurs, careful treatment is necessary to avoid further deterioration of the skin.

Of course, injury can cause a number of complications, depending on the nature, location, and severity of the injury. So do the best you can to protect yourself.

AN UNCOMPLICATED CONCLUSION

Don't spend all your time fretting about what's going to happen next. Enjoy your life, but always take care of yourself. This includes an awareness of the "state of your body."

19

Other Changes

We've discussed changes in your lifestyle that relate to taking care of your ostomy. But what about changes in other aspects of your life? One of your biggest concerns was probably that many changes would take place. However, there is one very positive thing to remember: once you have adjusted to the ostomy and to any necessary changes, very few long-lasting effects will be felt. "Great," you might say. "So, why do I feel so depressed?" Probably because, in the time immediately following surgery, you won't feel such optimism. Your head may be spinning, afraid of changes that may take place in your eating and bowel habits, traveling, working, social relationships, dealing with physical discomfort, to name a few. In fact, you may even be concerned that you won't be able to perform your normal chores and responsibilities. Time is a major intervening variable that can help you feel better. But realize that most ostomates feel this way at first. So if you are reading this section and know this is bothering you, realizing that you're not alone in feeling this way can help. Do you know what can help even more? Read this and smile: most of the people who feel this way initially *don't* feel this way after a while. Feelings improve. Being aware that you can do more certainly helps.

The rest of this book will address all of these concerns. The remaining chapters in Part III will be concerned primarily with changes in lifestyle related to things you do and the way your body feels.

20

Physical Changes

Caution: Reading this chapter may be hazardous to your health. Your emotional health, that is! Hazardous? Yes, if you start feeling that you have to change your life totally because of your ostomy. Read this chapter and learn about some of the potential changes. If there's anything you can do about them, suggestions will be offered. If not, at least you'll learn more about the changes. Most importantly, you'll learn that you're not alone in experiencing them. But remember—they may never happen.

Physical changes resulting from ostomy surgery do play a major role in the psychological adjustment to your new addition. You can't do something about all of them, but many of them can be helped. How? By changing things about yourself or your life. Even then, you may not be able to do anything about other changes. These you must learn to simply accept and live with, even if you don't like them. That may seem like a tall order, but what choice do you have? After all, you're still the same person inside (except for you-know-what). If there's nothing you can do, why not concentrate on those things you *can* do something about? Deal with any physical changes as they occur, one at a time. Don't anticipate the worst. How is that going to help?

There are a number of physical changes that may occur following surgery. Most of these may get better after a period of time. But be aware of the changes anyway, so that pessimism and depression do not set in if they occur.

FATIGUE

Fatigue (yawn!) is one of the more common results of any type of surgery, and is certainly no stranger to ostomates. Most people think of fatigue as negative. This is not always the case. It can be a positive. If you did not feel fatigued, you would push yourself too much! Then you'd certainly feel the effects, especially if it was immediately following surgery. What's the best way to cope with fatigue? Rest. (Clever!) A good night's sleep, or naps from time to time, are great for coping with fatigue. If you have experienced fatigue for long periods of time, you might want to check the nutritional make-up of your diet. Maybe it is not properly balanced (e.g. low blood sugar). Making changes in your diet may add to your energy.

Consider the possibility that your fatigue may be emotional rather than physical. In other words, you're tired because of the way you feel emotionally, not so much because of physical exhaustion. If this is the case, try to determine what emotional reactions are contributing to fatigue. Then you can work on improving them.

BODY TONE

A decrease in body tone is common following surgery. It's probably been a while since your muscles have been exercised (but hopefully not because you're lazy!). So what should you do? Obviously, the best answer is to exercise. However, do this only with your doctor's permission and get back into it slowly. Build up your body's condition gradually rather than forcing too much, too soon. Check with your physician to make sure that the activities you want to participate in will not interfere with your new condition. Certain muscles, for example, need to be tuned up so they will help intestinal activity. On the other hand, certain muscles that may have been weakened by surgery should not be pressed into service until healing is complete.

If you are going to exercise, be careful about perspiration. Perspiration decreases the fluid content of your body. You need to maintain a certain level of fluids. As an ostomate, you must be aware of any loss of electrolytes that may occur when you decrease your fluid level. Therefore, make sure that lost fluids are replenished. Drink lots! Water, Gatorade, and tomato juice are all very good for replacing fluids and electrolytes.

VISITS WITH OL' SOL

If you enjoyed sun-bathing before surgery, you don't have to necessarily restrict the amount of time spent in the sun now. But beware of the dangers of staying out too long. (Sunburn!) As an ostomate, you may have to consider any discomfort you may feel when wearing an appliance. If your appliance is of plastic or rubber, perspiration may cause irritation or discomfort. What do you do? Try wearing a pouch cover made from a soft, cottony material or fabric. This will absorb perspiration, rather than add to the sticky feeling.

REFRAIN FROM PAIN

One of the happiest physical changes resulting from ostomy surgery is the relief from prolonged pain due to illness. Since surgery may have been performed because of this pain, it is aimed at alleviating the pain. Many ostomates feel incredible relief and are able to live pain-free following recovery from surgery. If pain ever does creep into the picture, though, you'll certainly want to read the next chapter dealing with this miserable subject.

BODY APPEARANCE

One change that bothers many ostomates is an altered body appearance. This can be a result of the scars from surgery or from the stoma itself. Ileostomates or urostomates may be upset about a stoma that looks like a protruding nipple, sometimes extending almost an inch from the body. Fortunately, abdominal scars are rarely seen unless the skimpiest of bathing suits are worn. But this doesn't always help. Just knowing that the scars exist may make you unhappy.

So what should you do? If you are really upset about such scars, look into cover-ups or other cosmetic applications. Plastic surgery may even be considered in extreme cases. For the most part, however, not too much can be done about this. Does that mean it's hopeless? No. Keep telling yourself that it's good to be alive, and that people will accept you as you are. If you can learn to accept yourself, others will too. If some don't, who needs 'em?

WHAT ABOUT PHYSICAL RESTRICTIONS?

"What can't I do?" Or, better yet, "What *can* I do?" These are very important questions that you, as an ostomate, may ask. The answer? There is none. Every ostomate is different. There is no single activity that every ostomate should be told not to do. Here's a sensible thought. In the period of time following surgery, you shouldn't do any heavy abdominal activity, such as weightlifting! But once you've healed you should be able to participate in most normal activities. Often, parents are very restrictive with their children. They're afraid that they will be doing too much. So you'll probably have to restrict physical activities initially because of surgery. Eventually, though, you'll be able to participate in virtually any activity you choose. This does not mean that, if you were not very athletic before surgery, you should try out for the Olympics now! The most important thing is for you to take the best care of your health, shape, and self-esteem. Include activities that will ensure progress in each of these areas. Where children are concerned, improving self-esteem is very important. Those activities that lead to the child's feeling best about himself should be emphasized.

WHAT ABOUT WORKING?

Are you concerned about working? You really shouldn't be. If you are able to participate in physical activities, then you can work. The problem is that you may not feel like you can return to your old job. Maybe you're afraid that your employer doesn't want you or that you won't be able to get a new job. If this is a concern, or if you feel that there are medical or physiological restrictions, it might be a good idea to look into vocational rehabilitation. This can help you to learn new skills and create new possibilities for employment.

What about filling out job applications? Should you answer "yes" to questions asking if you have a physical disability? Most experts in the field of ostomy suggest that the answer is "no," since an ostomy is not a disability or handicap. It is simply something that is a part of you. Unless you are an individual who needs to be completely open and honest about your ostomy, there is no reason for you to volunteer any more information than you have to. This does not mean that you are lying or falsifying an application. Ethically, the only answers you must honestly provide are to questions about whether you've been hospitalized or had surgery. Even then, you can always indicate that you'll be glad to provide any additional information at a face-to-face interview. In this way, the prospective employer will see that you're "alive and kicking!"

A PHYSICAL FINALE

How can you help yourself? Here are a few general guidelines to keep in mind.

- Be aware of how your body feels. How is it reacting to what you are doing? Act accordingly.

- Build on the talents and activities you can still enjoy (there'll be plenty of them!).

- Pamper yourself a little. Learn that you don't have to do everything for yourself. Accept help from others when necessary and don't push yourself to do anything you can't. But don't depend on others any more than you must. You *do* want to be confident that you're in control!

- Be more protective of yourself. Take good care of your skin and manage your ostomy properly. Follow the normal routines you have established to get the proper amount of sleep, exercise, and nutrition. Avoid contagious diseases, injuries, and infections.

Remember: *you* are the most important ingredient in the recipe for the successful adjustment to having an ostomy. Help yourself.

21

Exercise

Up, down! Left, right! Twist, turn! Good night!

Exercise is one of the most important therapeutic treatments for an ostomate. Despite its advantages, however, you should never begin any exercise program without your physician's approval.

WHY EXERCISE?

Exercise is as important for psychological well-being as it is for your body. Exercise gives you the feeling of being able to do something. It clears your mind and helps you to control some of the unpleasant emotional reactions that may occur from time to time. Emotions such as depression, anger, fear, and frustration can all be helped by exercising. Exercise can also help to control stress.

Exercise can build up your self-confidence. Because you may initially lose some of the good feelings about yourself due to surgery and the change in your body image, exercise can help to rebuild confidence in your body. Seeing improvement in your performance as a result of exercise can also build up self-esteem.

Exercise is also essential to keep your body trim. One goal of exercise is to firm up the abdominal muscles. Firm, firm, firm is better than flab, flab, flab! This is also important in helping with stoma maintenance and an efficient digestive system. It can also strengthen your appetite so that you'll eat goodies containing all the proper nutritional elements necessary for good health.

You can decide what type of exercise you'd like to try, based on the things you like to do. In this way, you can enjoy the activity in addition to feeling healthier and helping your body. But wait—don't these sound like the same reasons why anybody would choose exercise?

What exercise can you participate in, considering your condition? Two of the best exercises for ostomates are walking and swimming. Besides that? How about skiing, swimming, golf, baseball, running, dancing, bowling, bicycling, tennis, sailing, or jogging? As you can see, you'll never be bored! Even some rough contact sports, such as football, hockey, or gymnastics, are within limits for those ostomates who have their physician's approval and, of course, are interested in these physically-demanding activities.

Do you know what can be frustrating? When you first begin to exercise following surgery—*wow*, will you be out of shape! That's not a put-down. Abdominal muscles need time to firm up following ostomy surgery. So any kind of exercise should be approached gradually. The longer it's been since you've exercised, the slower your return should be.

22

Weight Changes
and Nutritional Needs

Food, glorious food! Do you like to eat? It's one of the great pleasures of life. Therefore, it's not surprising for ostomates to be concerned about changes in diet. The number-one goal for any ostomate is to eat a well-balanced diet. Does that sound strange? Actually, it should be the number-one goal for everyone!

The fact that you have had an ostomy does not mean that your nutritional needs have changed. Nor does it mean that you can't try something new. But be careful! The consequences may not always be as desirable as you would like. If your condition before surgery required special dietary considerations, these should be continued, unless your physician has decided that they are no longer necessary.

A proper diet ensures that we consume all of the necessary vitamins, minerals, or supplements. Surgery may, however, cause some changes in your normal diet. In some cases, foods that you previously enjoyed may have to be reduced in quantity or eliminated because of possible adverse effects. For the most part, though, the majority of changes are for the better! For example, you may now be able to eat a wider variety of foods, especially if you've had ostomy surgery for Crohn's disease or chronic ulcerative colitis. Before surgery, your diet was probably bland and restricted (in other words, boring!), as you tried to control the illness without surgery. Now that surgery has eliminated the problem, you should be able to eat more the way you did prior to the onset of your illness. Thank goodness! Watch out, Alka-Seltzer!

To Diet or Not to Diet

Most people with ostomies do not require special diets. If your doctor feels it would be helpful for you, however, he will probably put you on either a reducing diet, a salt-free diet, or a low-protein diet (or a combination of the three). Avoid fad diets because they're just *not* nutritionally sound. Your cells need a nutritionally-balanced diet to maintain proper growth.

Back to Basics

Meals should be regularly scheduled. This facilitates a smooth digestive flow through your body system. A common misconception is that avoiding meals will reduce the amount of discharge from the stoma. This is not true. The ostomy works, regardless of whether or not you eat, so eat regularly-scheduled meals. Experiment carefully to see what foods agree with you. You may find that certain foods are more difficult for ostomy management. For example, if you are attempting to regulate waste elimination, certain foods may help and others may hurt. You'll learn by trial-and-error. Experience will teach you what foods to eat.

The specifics of a balanced diet are really beyond the scope of this book. For further information, consult a professional or go to the library. There are many excellent books that can give you all the details necessary to make sure your diet is balanced. However, if you've always been healthy and have eaten properly, there is no reason to believe that this will change.

If you find that a particular food disagrees with you, does this mean that it's gone forever? Not necessarily. You may be sensitive to a particular food at a particular time. You may want to try it again in another week or so to determine whether it was the food that caused the problem, or perhaps something else in your diet or environment. Emotional reactions may also cause different reactions to food. Eating a particular food at a different time, when you are in a different emotional state, may change its effect.

Adding Fiber (To your Diet, Not your Clothing)

Among the most important components of diet for anybody, especially the ostomate, is bulk or fiber. If you're a colostomate, adding fiber can be a natural way to regulate bowel activity. If you're an ileostomate, you must be careful not to include too much fiber. How much? This depends on how much intestine you have left. Want to improve the fiber content of your diet? Include bran. Bran can be eaten with cereal or in the form of muffins. It is usually a good idea to consume two to three tablespoons daily. Always check with your physician to make sure that these suggestions are appropriate for you, or to get additional ideas. Read any of the good books on fiber in your local library. In addition to the natural bulk of properly-balanced diets, there are supplements that can be taken. Certain tablets may increase the bulk content of waste material. The fiber contained in certain foods or in the "bulking" tablets adds more substance to the waste material. As a result, the muscle action of peristalsis works more efficiently.

Although fiber is very important, too much can be harmful. Too much fiber increases the chance of blockage, which is a problem you'll definitely want to avoid. Certain high-fiber foods, such as celery, coleslaw, popcorn, regular corn, Chinese vegetables, coconut, grapefruit, or other nuts, may be high in fiber and need to be restricted. This is especially true if you're an ileostomate. Colostomates and urostomates have very few food restrictions, if any.

Chew, Chew, Chew!

Make sure you chew all food thoroughly and completely. You've probably been hearing that since you were a kid! But it has added significance for an ostomate. In some cases (especially for ileostomates), foods that are not chewed well may appear at the other end in virtually the same forms as when they went in! Such items as corn, for example, may reappear in almost the identical shape and color. If this occurs, you're not doing the job, and it's barely being digested at all. In addition to corn, small foods such as peas or beans may be swallowed whole. If that happens, you're more likely to experience the joys of gas or irregularity of movement.

Odor

As we discussed in the sections on odor and gas, the foods you eat can add to the problem. Certain vegetables, for example, can be odor-causing.

Root vegetables, such as asparagus or parsnips, are on the "foul" list, as well as foods from the cabbage family, the legume family, prunes, eggs, onions, chicken, cheese, fish, beans, and even alcohol. This doesn't necessarily mean that such foods must be eliminated from your diet if you like them. But be aware of the possibilities, so that you can take extra precautions. You will learn what foods create problems for you and the best way to handle them. Some foods can be helpful in controlling or reducing odor! Parsley is one of the most beneficial foods. Not only is it tasty and leaves your mouth feeling fresh, but it also acts as a natural deodorant. It can help to control odor problems. Other green leafy vegetables, buttermilk, and yogurt can also help. For urostomates, drinking at least two glasses of cranberry juice daily, as well as taking Vitamin C tablets, can be very helpful in changing alkaline urine to that which is more acidic. Alkaline urine is dangerous because it builds up crystallized or alkaline salts on the inside of the appliances and around the opening of the stoma. This can be irritating and can cause stomal or skin excoriation.

This Section Is All Wet

A very important nutrient that is frequently overlooked is water. All ostomates should drink plenty of water, especially ileostomates. In this way, enough water is absorbed into the body to replace the water lost through the stoma. Remember that the large intestine is gone, so water absorption is decreased drastically in the intestinal tract. Water containing electrolytes simply passes out of the stoma. Say goodbye to the important substances that would normally be absorbed into the body through the large intestine. Some nutrients are absorbed in the small intestine. However, we can't afford to have the electrolytes pass out of the body through the stoma rather than be absorbed, or have potassium and other chemicals as well pass out of the body. But aren't there dangers from drinking a lot of water? Not to worry. Increasing your fluid intake will not soften the consistency of the waste material. If more water is consumed, more water will be absorbed. The amount that passes out through the stoma remains relatively the same. Drinking more fluids is helpful in flushing out the kidneys, eliminating impurities in the blood, and helping you to maintain the proper electrolyte balance.

What Are Electrolytes?

Electrolytes are electrical charges that exist in the body. They play a large role in determining how well the body functions. These electrolytic charges come from the digestion of certain foods, because these are the foods that contain necessary minerals. Can you guess what they are? Potassium is a primary one, along with calcium and sodium. Sodium is usually not as much of a problem as potassium because most people eat foods that already have more salt than they need. So even if some salt is lost through the stoma, other salt has already been absorbed. But normal diets are not as rich in potassium or calcium. The result? Deficiencies. Be sure to take in the proper amounts of these substances. And make sure that you're getting all the nutrients you need in adequate amounts.

There are foods that can help you to maintain proper levels of these nutrients. Foods rich in potassium and other necessary substances include bananas, prunes, oranges, and tomatoes. Because it is so important to maintain a proper fluid and electrolyte balance, you should also know what types of liquids to drink. Among the best are soups, fruit juices, shakes, coffee, iced tea, Gatorade, soda (such as Tab), ice cream, and even jello. Milk may not be too desirable, especially for those individuals who are lactose intolerant or for those who have higher levels of mucous or phlegm in the intestinal tract.

Does this mean that all fluids are wonderful? The specific fluids that you drink determine what other effects they may have. Alcoholic beverages, for example, may have good fluid content, but may have unique side effects (need I say more?). Carbonated drinks may cause gas or odor problems. Anybody could have these problems, but because of your ostomy they may be even more difficult to control.

This Section Is Heavy

Are you eating less now, and enjoying it less? Some ostomates experience a reduction in appetite. Along with this may come a desired (or undesired) weight loss. However, not everybody with an ostomy experiences this. Some people tend to eat more, and the pounds may increase effortlessly. Weight changes may occur as a result of surgery. The loss of your intestines or urinary tract, prolonged exposure to the wonders of hospital food, illness, chemotherapy, and other factors are among the reasons why you might lose weight during the time immediately prior to or following surgery. For someone who needed to lose some weight, this may be the cloud's silver lining. But don't put all the blame on your ostomy. Your weight may increase or decrease, and your appetite change; yet this fluctuation may have nothing to do with your ostomy. But maybe your weight is fluctuating because of weekend binges! Maybe you've gone to some food orgies! Perhaps you're retaining water (an *abused* excuse!), or maybe emotional crises have caused you to overeat. One of the most important things you can do to stay as healthy as possible is to eat properly and keep your weight at a proper level. Don't be a "junk-food junkie," unless you really have control over your eating habits.

Regardless of the reason for weight change, you'll still want to stabilize your weight at as close to your ideal weight as possible. Therefore, you'll want to control the number of calories you consume. Bulky food may be a problem. Many of these foods, useful in helping to move waste material along properly and controlling expulsion, may be fattening! Normally, if you were trying to diet, you'd probably cut out starches (all the goodies!). But if you do that as an ostomate, you may find that your bowel movements are less formed. With professional advice, it might be best to work out some sort of compromise. You may want to attempt a slower weight loss, but do it in a way that still keeps some firmness-controlling bulk in your diet. If you can handle this, weight changes should not be any more of a problem for you than for someone else. You know that you can exercise, and most activities are acceptable. Since eating and exercise are the two most important components of any weight-control program, you're in pretty much the same position as anyone else.

One reason why it is so important to control weight is because an excessive change in weight, either an increase or decrease, can alter the fit of your appliance. This can create other problems as well. If you want to lose weight, do so gradually. Just be aware of any changes in the way your appliance fits.

The Hard vs. The Soft of It

Constipation may be a bigger problem for colostomates than for ileostomates, because the amount of working intestine available for the absorption of water is longer. Constipation can be alleviated, if necessary, by consuming more of the foods that loosen waste. Which ones? Foods such as fruits, vegetables, fruit juices, and cereal fiber can "soften the problem."

On the other hand, diarrhea may be a problem for either the colostomate or the ileostomate. Diarrhea is dangerous if it occurs too often. You don't want to become dehydrated. Dehydration is especially a problem for ileostomates, since there is even less time for fluids to be absorbed by the body. A physician should be contacted if diarrhea persists. What foods can cause diarrhea? If you're having a problem, avoid milk and all milk products, raw fruits, very spicy foods, vegetables, and beer, among other things. Prunes may not be a good food to include in your diet. Can you guess why?! But there are some foods that may help to control diarrhea! Try apples, applesauce, rice, milk (that has been boiled), tapioca, peanut butter, bananas, or jello. Whew!

More on Dehydration

Because dehydration is such a problem, it must be avoided as much as possible. The best way to avoid it is obviously to increase your intake of fluids. Any ostomate, especially a child, should drink from four to eight glasses of liquids (non-alcoholic, please!) a day. Being thirsty is not necessarily an indication of dehydration. So don't think that, if you're not thirsty, you're not dehydrated. Physicians feel that thirst comes when dehydration has already occurred.

MEDICATION

Some people welcome medication as a powerful way to help their bodies. Others are afraid of its power, and of eventually becoming dependent on it. Still others resent having any artificial substances in their bodies. Where do you fit in? Your physician may believe that certain medication can be helpful to you, not necessarily for your ostomy specifically, but for any other problems that are part of your life.

Because of the chemical nature of medication and the way it may interact with your body, it is extremely important to follow your doctor's orders in taking the drugs prescribed for you. Do not play around with medication that hasn't been prescribed for you (or, as a matter of fact, even with that which has been prescribed!). Make sure you understand exactly why you are taking the medication, and what it is supposed to do.

How Do You Feel About Taking Medication?

This still doesn't mean you'll be thrilled with the idea. Not too many people are. What might your main concern be? You're probably concerned about what the medication may be doing to your body, or what the side effects may be. However, here's an interesting thought. Although no one cherishes the thought of experiencing side effects from a particular medication, at least side effects show you that the drug is potent. It's working! Hopefully, it will have an impact on the symptoms it is trying to alleviate.

You may experience certain emotional reactions (such as depression or anger), which must be dealt with (refer back to the chapters dealing with your emotions). Remember: if it is really necessary for you to take medication, you might as well let it do what it's supposed to. Accept it and don't let it bother you.

Taking Medicine

Let's say that you have to take certain medication. If so, try to take it in a form that is easy to digest. Why? Unless the medication is easily digested, and therefore absorbed quickly, it will pass through the body and out. You won't gain much benefit that way. This is especially true if you're an ileostomate. You're probably better off not using such medication as time-release capsules or medicine that comes in coated tablets or pills, since these may be expelled in almost the same form as they were taken. When they are working, they usually dissolve and are absorbed in the colon. If the colon has been removed, there is little chance of absorption. Therefore, it would probably be a good idea to take medication in liquid form.

AN ORAL FAREWELL

Please remember that all of the specific foods mentioned, as well as nutritional and medication needs, are only general suggestions. Each person is unique and will respond in a unique way. Only by learning about yourself, and experimenting with foods or beverages (under supervision, please), will you become aware of what's best for you.

23

Pain

Ouch! (Just getting you ready for this chapter!) Are ostomies painful? Fortunately, for the most part, no. Most ostomates feel little or no discomfort of any type once healing is complete. Obviously, post-surgical pain may occur, as it might for any other type of abdominal surgery. But the good news is that the most significant changes in pain are usually in a positive direction. If you previously suffered from Crohn's disease or ulcerative colitis, for example, pain relief after surgery will be a blessing.

One situation in which you might experience discomfort would be if you've had surgery that included the removal of your rectum. Once post-surgical pain has disappeared, rectal pain is known as the "phantom rectum" syndrome. This was mentioned in the chapter, *Problems or Complications*.

But back to the good news. For the most part, you shouldn't experience much, if any, pain following recuperative healing from surgery. But what if you do? How can you cope with any discomfort you might experience? The best way to cope with pain is to get rid of it! To do this, it's first necessary to identify the cause of the pain. Once this is done, treatment can be aimed at eliminating the cause. But there's a problem. In some cases, it may be impossible to do anything about the underlying source of pain. Therefore, the pain itself, rather than the cause of the pain, is the most important concern. Then what does treatment aim to accomplish? Relief from pain!

Where do you start? First, be aware of your pain. While this may sound strange, you'll learn to recognize whether your pain is something you can (and should) handle yourself, or if it is so serious that it needs to be attended to by a doctor. Remember: if in doubt, check it out. Discuss the pain with your doctor. Together you can work out the best ways of dealing with it.

MEDICAL TREATMENT

Medical treatment for pain generally involves medication. This can very effectively control a lot of problems, thereby ending the pain. For example, aspirin has been proven effective in controlling minor pain. But sometimes discomfort can continue, despite the use of medication. In extreme cases, further surgery may be helpful in treating the cause of the pain. But not all conditions lend themselves to surgical treatment. So it may be necessary for you to learn how to cope with some pain, rather than expect your physician to always relieve you of your discomfort.

ALLEVIATING THE PAIN

Is pain purely physiological? Rarely. It's usually a combination of physiological and psychological factors. What does this mean? Although there may be something in your body that is hurting, it is your mind that determines how much it hurts.

Lana was moving very slowly, primarily because she had a lot of rectal pain. The pain overwhelmed her every time she tried to move faster. Even when she was doing something she enjoyed, her movements were restricted. Suddenly, she heard her 9-year-old son cry out for help. Without thinking about her rectal pain, she went flying across the house to help him. This couldn't be purely physiological pain! Yes, Lana was in pain, but her mind probably magnified it greatly. When she realized her son was in trouble, she temporarily forgot about her pain.

What does all this mean? If medication or other medical intervention doesn't help alleviate your pain, you can still relieve some, if not all, of it by working on your mind's awareness of it. Read on to find out how you can do this.

Imagery

There is a relationship between your mind and the way you feel physically. Much research has proven this. Scientists have also found that bodily functions, previously thought to be totally beyond conscious control (autonomic is the medical term), can be modified using psychological techniques! One such technique is imagery, or the process of conjuring up pictures or scenes in your mind. In practice, imagery has been beneficial in helping to deal with a host of physiological and psychological problems, including headaches, hypertension, depression, and pain. In many cases, imagery procedures have worked well in combination with prescribed medication in treating illness.

This is how imagery works. Sit in a comfortable chair or in bed and get into a relaxed position. Lights should be dimmed, and outside sounds or noises minimized, with no interruptions. Breathe smoothly and rhythmically, allowing your body to release tension and relax. Then imagine a scene that you have chosen, trying to make the image as vivid and real as possible. This scene can be used therapeutically to help you feel better.

Doreen was suffering from painful headaches. She was instructed to relax and then develop an image of what the headache looked like. She imagined it as a very tight rubber band stretched around her head. Another person might imagine his or her head in a clamp. Whatever image you develop, it should be as vivid and detailed as possible. Doreen was then instructed to reverse what was happening in the image: she imagined the rubber band losing its elasticity. As a result, it became looser and looser around the head, and finally fell off. This allowed the head to relax and eliminated discomfort.

You may want to use imagery to reduce rectal pain. Images you could use include oil being squeezed into the area, a soothing lotion being applied to the affected area, or a warm bath. These images can be used anywhere. (Have you ever taken a bath in a bus?!) With regular use, they can help you feel better. Imagery is really only restricted by your creativity. A good book on the subject is *In The Mind's Eye*, by Arnold Lazarus. See if your public library or local bookstore has it.

Biofeedback

Biofeedback combines the procedures of relaxation and imagery with the use of measuring instruments, usually electronic. The machines let you know what's going on physiologically (giving you *feedback*) in your body (*bio*). The devices, which are connected to different parts of your body, give you moment-by-moment information about any changes that are taking place.

Gayle was experiencing a lot of abdominal pain, so her physician suggested she try biofeedback. A machine measuring muscle tension was attached to her abdomen (in much the same way that electrodes from an EKG machine are connected. There is *no* pain, and you won't get jolted!) As she attempted to relax her abdominal muscles, the machine gave her instant feedback as to whether she was really relaxing the muscles, and to what degree. As she became aware of her lowering tension, she learned what mental images were helping her to relax. She could then continue using these images on her own, without the machine, to help her relax and control some of the pain.

What kinds of biofeedback equipment may be used? Most frequently, machines can be used to measure skin temperature, pulse, blood pressure, the electrical activity resulting from muscular tension, or electrical activity coming from the brain.

Coping Psychologically

There are other factors that can contribute to the intensity (even the very existence) of your pain, including your emotional state, the attention you pay to it, and the way the rest of your body feels. Obviously, as you pinpoint which of these factors does play a role, you can begin improving the way you cope with pain.

You'll want to do everything you can to decrease fear, stress, tension, and other emotional factors. All of these may make you more aware of your painful physical state. Anything you can do to relieve anxiety and tension (including psychotherapy, if necessary) should help you to cope better with any pain.

How do you reduce the amount of attention focused on your pain? Of course, the more time you have to think about it, the worse it will seem. So try to divert your attention. Develop other interests that require concentration. Of course, how well you do depends on how much you can do.

AN UNAGONIZING CONCLUSION

If you ever do have any pain, whether from the ostomy or from something else, don't throw in the heating pad! Realize that the pain will not last forever. A lot can be done, both medically and psychologically, to help deal with it.

24

Clothing

What kind of "clothes horse" were you prior to surgery? Did you like fashionable, stylish clothes, or were you willing to cover your body with whatever was available? Do clothing concerns really matter to you?

A depressing thought you may have after surgery is that you'll always have to wear loose-fitting, uninteresting clothes. Even if you were a sloppy dresser before surgery, you may still lament the fact that you can't wear the nice clothes everyone was telling you to wear! But fear not. It doesn't stay this way. Fortunately, as time goes on, the only ostomates who actually wear these loose-fitting garments are those who really want to! You will be able to indulge in all kinds of stylish clothing. As you heal from surgery, your stoma will decrease slightly in size, as the puffiness and swelling go away. As you become more confident in taking care of your stoma, you will find that you're able to wear tighter-fitting clothing. This type of clothing obviously should not be restrictive, but it can certainly be more form-fitting and flattering than you may have originally thought. As time goes by, you'll find that there will be few, if any, clothing restrictions.

"FRINGE" BENEFITS

Wearing nice clothes has always been a very good way to help your self-image. You'll feel more cheerful when you dress nicely. Having to wear baggy clothing could certainly affect your self-image. This may be one of the reasons for feeling "down" after surgery. But as you feel better, and you're again able to wear nice-looking, stylish clothes, you'll feel good and look good. Your self-image will improve as well. You may even feel better by just going out and buying new clothes.

MOVE GRADUALLY

Should you rush out and purchase designer originals? No. Take it easy. Buying new clothes should be delayed until you've completely recovered from surgery, the size of your stoma has stabilized, and tenderness in your abdomen has, for the most part, disappeared. Don't rush. You've got time. Although your stoma size may remain the same, you may still experience abdominal tenderness. Initially you may want to wear more loosely-fitted clothing, just to be comfortable. But this doesn't mean that your clothing has to be sloppy or unstylish.

Sleep-wear may change as a result of ostomy surgery as well. You may feel more comfortable in nightgowns or nightshirts than pajamas, especially if you toss and turn during the night. If you wear clothing with elastic bands, you may want to modify it so that the elastic does not rest on your stoma or on another tender area.

Once you completely recover from surgery, you'll have very few restrictions. Even the snuggest-fitting clothing can be worn comfortably, as long as it does not cause a problem for your stoma. You might worry about tight clothing interfering with the functioning of your appliance. But again, fear not! Appliances have come a long way in recent years. As long as they fit properly, and you use caution in placing pressure directly on the opening, you should have few problems. It is less likely that appliances will be noticed even when you wear more form-fitting clothing. Appliances have been designed so that they can even be worn under bathing suits that leave little to the imagination!

WHAT ABOUT KIDDIES?

The clothing needs of children with ostomies don't have to be any more elaborate than they might otherwise be. After healing from surgery, children can wear just about anything they like. Dungarees, baseball uniforms, bathing suits, shorts—all are perfectly acceptable. Obviously, parents will want to get clothing that requires minimal care. In this way, if any problems do arise, it will be easier to take care of them.

A FASHIONABLE FINALE

Initially, you'll probably fear that fashion will no longer be much of a pleasure. Gone are the days when modern-looking clothes could be worn, tailor-fitted and attractive-looking. In order to protect the stoma, the appliance, and yourself from the stares of strangers, you may feel that you'll have to wear bulky clothing to hide what lies on your abdomen from the world. But it's not going to be like this. You can dress nice, look nice, and feel nice. It's only a matter of time.

25

Financial Problems

Having an ostomy can be a pain, and not just a pain in the gut. Having an ostomy can be a pain in the pocketbook! It can be expensive. The expense revolves around the medical costs, the cost of regular checkups, as well as the costs of the appliances and other necessary equipment. The cost varies considerably for each ostomate. Some people estimate the cost of managing an ostomy to start at as little as $150 or $175 a year, depending on the equipment used and the frequency of appliance changes. The cost of ostomy management in children is usually higher because children wear appliances for shorter periods of time. Since they must be changed more often, more cost is involved.

INSURANCE CAN BE AN ASSURANCE

Insurance coverage is essential. For ostomates, certain costs may be reimbursable by third-party payments. Insurance companies do cover medical costs. However, contrary to what may go on in other countries, insurance companies may not cover the cost of appliances or equipment. Medicare, Medicaid, and other services, such as Crippled Childrens' Services, may be helpful in defraying some of the costs.

But what happens if you run out of money or insurance, or if your coverage is not good enough? Even worse, what if you can't get insurance? Because you have an ostomy, you may have more difficulty getting it, whether it be life insurance or health insurance. However, you should not be discriminated against because of your ostomy. On the other hand, some ostomates find that they are eligible for even more benefits than they originally thought. The best rule of thumb is to speak to a reputable insurance agent and find out exactly what you are entitled to.

WORK OR HOME

Financial problems arise from lost earnings or income. Following surgery, you won't be able to work at all. Later on, maybe you still won't be able to go back to work, or maybe you can only hold down a part-time job. Perhaps your "employability" will be reduced because of your ostomy. (It shouldn't be, but you can't always convince employers.)

An ostomy can also be costly because of changes at home. You may need outside help as you recover. Maybe you'll need a babysitter for your children, or a cleaning woman. All of these things cost money, adding to your financial burden. Therefore, dealing with financial problems because of your ostomy can certainly be distressful. As your medical costs rise, your budget becomes tighter and tighter. If costs continue to skyrocket, you may feel like you're being strangled!

CAN ANYTHING HELP?

Before you do anything, talk to people. Find out what others have done. How do you find them? Ask your physician or E.T. for suggestions, or contact your local chapter of the Ostomy Association. Speak to others in similar situations to find out how they handle their money problems. Even though you may initially be embarrassed to bring up the subject, the common bond that exists among people with an ostomy tends to smooth this over quickly. You'll be glad you brought it up.

If medical costs are overwhelming you, consider attending a clinic. Because clinics usually operate on a sliding-scale fee schedule, you may be able to get quality medical care at a reduced cost. In some cases, you may even see the same physician you'd normally see, since many physicians graciously donate their time to clinics.

A very important source of financial support is insurance coverage. There are some government insurance programs that you might find helpful. Let's discuss these different government programs, what they do, and how you can participate (if you're eligible).

Before we do, there is one important thing to remember. In general, ostomy surgery does not result in disability. However, certain underlying conditions that may have contributed to the need for surgery may be (or have been) disabling. Speak to someone familiar with the rules. Don't apply unless you really have a good case. Otherwise, it's a waste of time. Many people get turned down even though they deserve benefits. Consider other forms of financial support.

Social Security (Disability)

The Social Security Disability Program is a Federal Government Program. It is administered and run by the Social Security Administration. The money that funds the Social Security Benefit Plan comes from workers and their employers. Because of this, one of the main requirements for receiving benefits is that you must have worked for five out of the ten years prior to your disability. However, if you became disabled before turning 31, the five-year requirement is reduced to one and a half years. In other words, if Olivia Outofdough, age 28, wanted to receive disability benefits, she would only have to prove that she worked for eighteen months during the previous ten years. However, if Olivia was lying (to herself and the government) about her age and was actually 38, she'd then have to prove five years of work experience in the past ten.

Benefits are available from the Social Security Disability Program to those of you who fit into the following categories:

1. Individuals under 65 who are disabled (and their families).

2. Single individuals under the age of 22 who were disabled before that age and are still disabled.

3. Widows who are disabled.

4. Widowers who are disabled and also dependent.

There are also other specific cases that may entitle you to benefits.

There is one very rigid rule that the Social Security Administration enforces in order for benefits to be approved. This guideline is: "The physical or mental impairment must prevent you from doing any substantial, gainful work, and is expected to last (or has lasted) for at least 12 months, or is expected to result in death." In other words, it is expected that your disability prevents you from doing any meaningful work. This must be the case if you are applying for disability benefits.

Once you meet the eligibility requirements for disability benefits, does this mean that cash will start pouring in? Not so fast! There are still other steps that you have to go through. You will have to provide the names and addresses of people involved in treating you, including physicians, hospitals, or clinics. Medical records must be provided, substantiating the dates and treatments prescribed. This information will be evaluated by a Social Security team (including a physician), and additional tests may be required to support your claim.

Supplemental Security Income (SSI)

Once you apply for Social Security benefits, you also become eligible for Supplemental Security Income. This leads to eligibility for Medicaid. The Supplementary Security Income Program is also run by the Social Security Administration, which operates the Social Security Benefit Program. However, whereas Social Security benefits come from workers and their employers, SSI comes from a general treasury fund.

SSI benefits are available to individuals 65 and over, the blind, and the disabled. The requirements to receive SSI include the same definitions of disability that are used for Social Security benefits.

Medicaid

Medicaid is the more commonly-used term for Medical Assistance. Benefits are provided automatically for anyone who qualifies for Supplemental Security Income. Medicaid will cover virtually any medical-related expense, as long as you go to a professional who is a "participant provider." This provider is then directly reimbursed by the state for the service provided to you.

Medicaid applies if you are 65 or over and are receiving Social Security, or if you are under 65 and have met the Social Security requirements for disability. In addition, Medicaid is provided to families on welfare, and to children under age 21.

Medicare

In order to be eligible for Medicare benefits, you must have received disability checks for at least two consecutive years. This applies only if you are under 65, since Medicare benefits are provided to anyone 65 or over. Another acceptable criterion for receiving Medicare benefits is if you have permanent kidney failure, requiring dialysis or a kidney transplant.

Medicare is another part of the Social Security Administration. There are two components to the Medicare Program. The medical insurance component helps you to pay for physicians' services and out-patient services, including physical therapy and speech pathology, among others. The hospital insurance component covers in-patient care and nursing care within a facility.

Medicare benefits are limited and rigidly evaluated. They are only applied to charges that are deemed reasonable and necessary in treating your disease.

What Should You Do?

To determine whether or not any of these programs are applicable to you, contact your local Social Security office. In addition, consult your physician or your local support group. These sources should provide you with valuable information that will assist you in determining which programs can help you. But beware. These programs are strict. They are more eager (so it seems) to reject your claim than to accept it. You can appeal if your application is rejected, but this becomes even more aggravating. Want some advice? Talk to people who have been through it. Talk with members of your local Ostomy Association chapter. Fight for your rights, and for your dollars.

$UMMING UP

Although ostomies can be costly, there's still some hope. More and more people are learning about their costly impact. Hopefully, the variety of insurance coverages available to you will increase, more provisions will be made for meeting your expenses, and requirements and application procedures will become more "human."

26

Traveling

Ben was a 45-year-old business executive. One reason why he always enjoyed working hard at his job was because it provided him with an income sufficient to take his family on luxurious annual vacations. He and his family would spend many happy weeks in many different parts of the world. However, since undergoing ostomy surgery to resolve an intestinal problem, Ben had not taken any trips at all. In the 18 months following surgery he used every possible excuse to avoid going away because he was so afraid of being away from his "home base."

Does it have to be this way? Definitely not. Ostomates can go anywhere! Frequently, ostomy surgery even increases your ability to travel. Why? You may be relieved of many of the restrictions that your previous condition imposed. This would make it easier for you to get away.

Do all ostomates avoid traveling? No. Some ostomates travel simply to prove to themselves that they can. This doesn't mean that there are no fears attached. But they do want to prove to themselves that they can do it, and that traveling, as one of life's pleasures, is possible. As with any other aspect of ostomy care, planning ahead and taking the proper precautions can allow you to travel with a free mind (although not with free airfare!) Let's explore some of the types of planning ahead you should do before a vacation.

TAKING SUPPLIES

One of your biggest concerns about traveling may be: what happens if I run out of sufficient supplies for my needs? There are two things you can do. First, have a sufficient number of extra supplies in case any un-expected situations arise. Second, be aware of whether or not you'll be able to find surgical supply houses where you're traveling. How do you do this? Look through the Yellow Pages for the area that you'll be visiting—that is, if it is a domestic city. Otherwise, speak to officials from any foreign country you might visit. You could contact the foreign embassy to find out if any such stores or ostomy organizations exist there.

Regardless of your success in finding surgical supply houses, you should still take extra appliances and supplies to meet virtually any need. If you are flying (in a plane!), take some changes of appliances and extra supplies with you for the flight. Do not pack all supplies in your luggage. There are two reasons for this. First of all, if your luggage ends up in Kalamazoo when you're flying to Dallas, you don't want to be left without what you need. Second, if you need to change appliances on the plane, it would be rather difficult for you to ask the flight attendant if you can climb down into the baggage hold to get these supplies! So always have a change available.

What should you carry with you? Other than changes in appliances, take large, plastic sandwich bags for disposal purposes. Carry tissues, toilet paper, or towelettes for cleaning. If necessary, take a small plastic bottle containing water for irrigating. Take extra clips for hanging irrigation equipment, or other needed paraphernalia. Take extra adhesive for the appliances. Some cautious travelers even take a large bath towel or sheet, with tape or thumb tacks, to set aside areas of privacy. For example, in some foreign countries, public restrooms have stalls without doors. You might not be too thrilled about changing or emptying an appliance in such a setting. You might even want to take "Do Not Disturb" signs (in the appropriate language!).

If you're on any medication, make sure that you have an adequate sup-ply. Even more importantly, make sure that you have spares in properly-labeled containers. You never can tell when you may lose some of your original supply. You may want to ask your physician to write up extra prescriptions to take with you. In case there is any reason for you to need more, you'll be prepared. If you're going to a foreign country, you may want the prescription translated into the language of that country, in case the pharmacist has difficulty understanding English.

Not only should you take extra supplies, but you should also have a list of all equipment and supplies that you need and the name of the manufacturer. If possible, the manufacturer's address and telephone number should also be included, so that in an emergency you can contact the manufacturer directly to order a quick shipment of materials.

IDENTIFY YOURSELF!

It's always a good idea to travel with complete identification, not just for your luggage but for yourself. The Medic Alert bracelet, indicating that you have a medical problem, is accepted worldwide as identification of a special need in physical health. In addition, make sure your wallet contains an identification card with complete information about your condition, the type of medication you may need, the type of appliances you use, whether or not you irrigate, and any other information pertinent to your condition. Again, if you're going to a foreign country, you might make sure that this information is translated into the language of that country. What if foreign languages were never your forte? Try checking with a teacher of that particular foreign language in a local school. Check with the airline that travels to that country. Representatives who speak the language would probably be willing to translate for you. As a last resort, you may want to check with the foreign embassy of that particular country. This may take a little extra time, but your mind will be more at ease when you do travel.

AIRPLANE ANTICS

Let's say your vacation is set, you're flying to Paradise, and you're now making final preparations before leaving for the airport. Any special considerations? You bet!

Anticipate the Pressure

If you are flying, beware of the pressure. Atmospheric pressure, that is! If you are carrying any tubes, droppers, or pressurized containers, remove as much excess air from these as possible. In this way, the change in air pressure as you go up will not cause any unpleasant surprises. How do you do this? Remove the cap or top and gently squeeze until all the air has been expelled. Then, while holding the tube or container in that position, replace the cap.

Inspection Time

If you are traveling by air, you may want to arrange to have your luggage inspected privately. This applies to luggage coming through customs at your foreign destination or back in the States, or to luggage containing extra supplies that you'll be taking on board. Private inspection avoids potential embarrassment and keeps the long lines moving.

If you don't want to trigger the alarm as you walk through the x-ray detector before getting on your plane, you may want to inform the security agent that you are carrying or wearing appliances containing metal parts. Metal detectors may suspect that you're trying to hijack the plane with your face plate! The alarm may be triggered, and you certainly don't want to be frisked! At the same time, do you really want to strip to show the security guard that you're not wearing a dangerous appliance? What should you do?

Bring an extra appliance with you. You can show it to the guard and explain that it's the same as what you are carrying or wearing. To be even more prepared, you may want to bring along a physician's note explaining the need for the appliance. These are extra precautions, certainly. But if you are a worried traveler, or you haven't been doing much, if any, traveling because of a number of fears, this is an additional means of reassurance. Also, please remember that it is rare that you would ever encounter this problem.

Eating on Board

If you have special dietary needs, you may want to check in advance to find out what food is being served on the plane. Most airlines know their menus in advance. If, however, you are flying cut-rate, you may be playing potluck with your meals. When in doubt, take some of your own food with you for the flight. You don't want a bad food reaction to start your vacation off on the wrong foot!

EATING ABROAD

Foreign eating and drinking occasionally cause problems for any traveler. Therefore, you really have to be on guard against and aware of potential problems. Unless you've been assured that it's o.k., don't drink tap water or even water in thermoses provided by hotels. Avoid fruits or vegetables that may have been washed before being served. Avoid any other foods that include water in their preparation. Even something as simple as brushing your teeth can make you wish you were back home in bed. You've heard of Montezuma's Revenge? Well, Montezuma has traveled to many parts of the world! The best way to conquer the water problem is to use pure, sterilized, or distilled water. This type of water should be used for irrigation as well. Some hotels will provide water purifiers so that you can take water from the tap, process it, and then be able to use it safely.

It is not always safe to even drink typical American soft drinks when abroad. The name of the soft drink may be American, and the packaging may look the same as it does in the United States, but that doesn't mean that it has been made in the U.S. If the drink was manufactured or even bottled locally, you still run some risks. Any foods you do eat should be well cooked and properly prepared. Avoid foods that do not look or smell the way you'd expect them to. It's better to be safe (and hungry) than full and uncomfortable.

If you do want to eat any fruits or veggies, peel them carefully, throw away the peels, and wash them with purified water. If any food has a broken skin or looks damaged, throw it away. You're usually better off not eating any foods that haven't been cooked. Canned baby foods that are available in large markets can be good dietary supplements (remember, you did like them once!). Here is a disappointing thought, however. Pastries, especially those made with cream, can be dangerous (and not just to your waistline). If they're not taken care of properly, bacteria can grow in them. As far as meats are concerned, be very careful where you eat and what you choose to eat. American laws are very strict about the inspection of meats served to the public. Laws may not be as strict or may even be nonexistent in other countries. Therefore, you run the risk of eating improperly-cooked meats, meats that have not been prepared appropriately, and so on. Use good judgment. You may ask, "Why can't I eat this when the people who live here eat it all the time?" Don't be jealous. You don't know if that's true. You don't know if they eat these foods or if they avoid them, too. Or maybe natives are used to these foods and their lead-lined stomachs can handle foods that your stomach can't. Maybe hundreds of natives are home in bed with food poisoning! At any rate, be sure to protect yourself.

Are you beginning to think that, because there is so much to be afraid of, you won't be able to enjoy your vacation? Don't feel that way. Just remember—you're not going on vacation merely to eat. (If you are, don't go someplace where food is such a problem!) Instead, try to emphasize the other, more enjoyable aspects of your trip. Adequate preparation and total awareness are easy to achieve and will certainly help to make your trip an enjoyable one. If, despite your preparations, you cannot success-fully regulate the way your body reacts and diarrhea results, you should certainly try to control it. Use medication, which you should always bring from home. Or, if the medication doesn't work, try foods such as rice, bananas, and crackers. In an emergency, try pure chocolate. But you may have to search for it, or bring some with you, because the chocolate in candy bars is not the pure type that can be helpful. Put a cork on diarrhea as quickly as possible. Don't just wait for it to stop because you then run the risk of dehydration. If you are unsuccessful in stopping it in a relatively short period of time, see a physician.

PREPARING FOR CARING

One chief concern you may have when traveling is where you can get proper medical care if necessary. So prepare for this, too. Compile a list of clinics, hospitals, and physicians in different parts of the world where you may be traveling. In addition, find out the locations of local chapters of ostomy associations. They can be of great support to you. There are hun-dreds of chapters of the United Ostomy Association in this country, and there are also chapters of the Association abroad. Check with your own local chapter to find out addresses. The winter issue of the *Ostomy Quarterly*, the regular publication of the United Ostomy Association, always contains a list of all the chapters within this country. This list can be helpful if you ever need a chapter at your disposal. Whether you need these facilities or not, knowing that you have their addresses will give you peace of mind.

What should you do if you're planning to go someplace where there are no appropriate facilities or physicians, or where they might be hard to find? You might consider going someplace else! If you decide that you want to go there anyway, and there are no facilities available, at least you're showing confidence in handling your situation. If you feel uncomfortable, on the other hand, don't go on vacation with this cloud hanging over your head. You're better off going someplace else. Other places can be equally exciting, and you'll be reassured to know that there are facilities for emergency needs. As a final measure, the American embassy in a foreign country will assist you in getting what you need.

WHAT ABOUT SLEEPING?

Are you reluctant to travel because you don't like the idea of sleeping in a strange bed? Maybe you're worried about accidents while you are sleeping. If you have any such concerns, bring some type of mattress cover with you. Even if it's as simple as a large plastic bag, it will help you to sleep peacefully without worrying about the consequences of an accident. Are you also uncomfortable about the idea of using strange bathrooms? Obviously, you don't want to be afraid of these things forever. Nor do you want to force yourself to live with them by going on this vacation. Gradually work at trying new things, even before your trip.

AUTOMOTIVE APPREHENSIONS

If you're traveling by car, don't eat too much. This will make it easier for you to ride in comfort and reduce the number of unscheduled pit-stops. Carry a pitcher, thermos, or cooler containing juices or any other goodies you'd like.

When you're sitting in the car, wear your seatbelt either above or below your stoma. This will help you to avoid excessive or prolonged pressure. If you stop to eat along the way, don't eat foods that are unusual or aren't a part of your normal eating plan. This is really not the best time to experiment.

A FINAL CONFIRMATION

Remember, not everyone is like Ben. Many ostomates feel absolutely no reluctance to travel anywhere. In many cases, when you get over the surgery, you may even be more willing and enthusiastic about traveling, and do more things than you have previously done.

If you haven't traveled since your surgery, you may want to build up your confidence by taking short trips first. If you have just finished recovering from surgery, taking a three-month trip around the world might be a bit much! Even an overnight trip might be traumatic. Start with a couple of day trips, then weekend trips, working your way up to short-distance, week-long excursions. Don't do all this within the first few months, of course! Expanding your travel activities slowly is a good way to develop your confidence.

A lot of information has been provided here—mostly precautionary, but nevertheless realistic and sensible. You may need extra time to prepare for your vacation (more time than the "average" traveler). However, with this extra preparation you should be able to enjoy a wonderful vacation, just as anybody else would. Don't forget to send me a postcard!

PART IV

Interacting with Other People

27

Coping with Others
—An Introduction

You do not live your life alone (unless you're reading this book on a deserted island in the Pacific). You interact with many people every day. One of the biggest problems for a new ostomate is anticipating difficulties in interpersonal relationships. What are others going to think? How are they going to react? Are they going to ask questions? What kinds of answers will they listen to and what kinds will turn them away? These are some of the questions that may bother you. Since dealing with other people comprises a majority of your waking hours, it is important to discuss how an ostomy can affect these relationships. Obviously, different problems can exist in different relationships. But before we begin discussing each type of relationship specifically, there are a few general points to be made.

DO UNTO OTHERS...

When you interact with others, you cannot become totally wrapped up in your own feelings. If you disregard the feelings of others, you'll also prevent them from getting close to you. You'll have to consider how others feel, just as you'd like them to consider your feelings. What does this mean? You're not the only one who has to cope with having an ostomy. Important people in your life are also having a hard time, simply because you mean a lot to them. Remember that. Some people tend to feel that their problems don't affect anyone else. "How can they feel upset? It's happening to *me!*" But is that fair? Take your family, for example. A problem for you is also a problem for your family. Of course, it may be affecting you differently from them. Maybe you're the one experiencing the apprehension and embarrassment, but it still affects the people who care about you. You'll be better able to cope with these important people, as well as help yourself to cope better, by remembering this.

YOU CAN'T CHANGE OTHERS

A major mistake you might make is to feel that if you try hard enough you can change the attitudes, feelings, or behaviors of others. It doesn't happen that way. Whether they accept your ostomy or deny that you have a problem at all, you can't change them. You can only change yourself. Spend more time working on *you*, and worry less about others. They may change, but it will more likely be a result of the changes they see in you. Help yourself. Be your own best friend.

LOOK THROUGH THE EYES OF OTHERS

If you have an argument with someone, you may believe that you're right and the other person is wrong. In this case, nothing will be resolved. Take a moment and look at the situation through the eyes of the other person. What does he or she see? What might the other point of view be? This will definitely help you to better understand the problem. If you look at it only through your own eyes, someone else's behavior may drive you crazy. Looking through the eyes of others can help you to better understand them and to improve your relationships with them. If you then try to have a discussion, this will also help you to explain how you feel.

PRIDE, YES! REVENGE, NO!

Revenge! There are times when you might think, "I only wish that _____ (insert appropriate name!) could know what it's like to live with an ostomy for an hour, a day, or a week, so that he/she could understand what I've been going through." But you know this isn't realistic, and you can't sit around waiting for it to happen. Besides, afterwards you might not be too pleased with yourself for having such vengeful thoughts. So what should you do? Take pride in yourself. Concentrate on doing what's best for *you*. If you have to be a little more self-centered and a little less concerned about what other people think, just accept this as one more way of coping with your ostomy.

A LITTLE SELFISHNESS IS O.K.

What happens if you're feeling rotten, but others want you to keep doing more and more? In the past, you may have had trouble saying no, because you'd either feel guilty or you didn't want to disappoint someone or hurt their feelings. But now you must curtail your generosity because it can hurt you. Frequently, you may have to give the appearance of being selfish. Do for yourself; think of yourself. You're Number 1, and that's the way it must be. If you take care of yourself, then you can be in the best shape to deal with others. The reverse does not hold true. If you are best for others, you may not be best for yourself.

BRING ON THE WORLD

Now that we've started with some general ideas, let's see how an ostomy can affect different relationships you may have with people. Of course, not every chapter will apply to you. You can either read the chapters that are appropriate for you, or read them all and realize that different kinds of problems do exist in any relationship.

28

Your Family

Blood is thicker than water! Your family can be a critical factor in your successful adjustment to having an ostomy. Why? You're probably with your family more than with anyone else. If you get along well with members of your family, you'll have a solid foundation from which to move towards a triumphant adjustment to other factors.

A common concern in dealing with family members is how to handle their curiosity about seeing your abdomen and stoma. You may be uncomfortable about this. You may feel like you're exposing yourself. But if you do decide to share, this can help them to understand your new addition. You'll probably feel better after they've seen it. One of your fears may be the fear of rejection by anyone who sees your ostomy. Your self-image may have suffered, and you may fear that loved ones may be turned off by what they see. However, if family members express curiosity, you may want to get it over with. This doesn't mean that you have to walk down Main Street with your belly exposed so that there's no more mystery! You're only thinking about sharing this with your family—people who are close to you. "Do I have a choice?" you might wonder. Of course you do. You don't have to "bare all!" If you decide not to, it's o.k. Tell yourself that it's not necessary to show anyone your stoma and appliance. Just play each situation by ear. You'll make the right decision.

ALL IN THE FAMILY

There are various types of problems that may pop up with different members of your family. So let's discuss how to cope with each specific member of the family.

COPING WITH YOUR SPOUSE

Of course, have an ostomy has a definite effect on yor marriage. But this doesn't mean that problems can't be resolved. Through better communication, understanding, and counseling (if necessary), there are very few problems that can't be worked out. Let's discuss some of the ways in which a marriage may feel the impact of ostomy surgery.

Social Life Changes

Have you decided to cut back on your social activities because of your ostomy? For any of the reasons discussed in previous chapters (regardless of whether they're valid or not), you may temporarily feel the need to curtail some of the activities that you used to enjoy with your spouse. This can be hard to bear, especially if you both had active social lives before your surgery. Because your spouse does not have an ostomy, he or she may feel anger, frustration, or helplessness. Take comfort in the fact that, as you get better, you can get out again. If, however, your social life is still on hold even after you've recovered from surgery, you'll have to ask yourself if this is due to certain fears or apprehensions. If so, refer to other appropriate chapters (such as *Fears and Anxieties*) for suggestions and support.

If Family Responsibilities Must Change . . .

Your ostomy may create a need for temporary or permanent changes in each family member's responsibilities. This is another potential source of friction between you and your spouse, especially when your spouse receives a heavy share of the load. "Re-assigning" chores to different members of the family can be very difficult for all.

Mary Lou, a 31-year-old mother of two, used to make lunch for her husband and children each morning. Now, with the added responsibility of ostomy maintenance, she no longer had time before they left for work or school. (She also refused to get up an hour earlier!) So she "transferred" this responsibility to her husband. Since he had difficulty boiling water, he wasn't too thrilled. He, in turn, placed added responsibilities on the children. This created even more tension. Despite the fact that Mary Lou's family loved her and was concerned about her health, they were all understandably upset, especially her husband. How can you change things as smoothly as possible? Make changes gradually. The ability to afford household help will make things easier, of course. But regardless of this, try to avoid overwhelming your spouse. Be realistic in your expectations.

How else can you help your spouse to adjust to greater burdens? Make sure free time is still available for the pleasures in life. It's only when the new responsibilities seem to be all-consuming that serious problems may occur. As always, look at these changes through the eyes of your spouse. Consider how you'd feel if the situation were reversed. Think how upsetting it would be if you no longer had time for things you enjoyed because of added responsibilities and pressures. Discuss it reasonably, and be gentle.

Denial

What do you do if your spouse simply won't accept the fact that you have an ostomy? You might hear, "Come on, everything's the way it was. What's the big deal?" This is tough to swallow. You can try to "educate" your spouse, but you mustn't overdo it. If you're constantly badgering, reminding your spouse of the things that have changed because of the ostomy, you certainly won't convince someone who has obviously been denying its very existence. Your spouse will not accept your ostomy until ready to do so. Concentrate on your own feelings. Don't feel that you have to flaunt your stoma before your spouse, or in front of anyone else who doesn't accept it. Feelings may change, but slowly.

In Sickness and in Health? Sorry!

Unfortunately, some marriages have ended because of ostomies. Former feelings of closeness and intimacy may be replaced by the unwelcome feelings of coldness and distance. Some spouses have so much difficulty accepting changes in appearance and behavior that the "magic" seems to fly out of the marriage. And it may not be all your spouse's fault. You may be so apprehensive that you can't enjoy your relationship. Your sensitivity may cause you to be less patient. So marital breakups *do* occur. But realize that about 50% of all marriages end in divorce anyway, even when no ostomies are involved!

Statistics aside, what do you do if your spouse is frightened and "wants out?" Your spouse's fear, your own condition, and your fears of abandonment all combine to create a horrible package of anxiety, depression, hopelessness, and panic. This package isn't one you can (or should) handle alone and, at this point, you probably won't be able to talk to your spouse. You may find communication with your spouse either nonexistent or destructive. Get some help. Seeking the aid of a professional or an objective outsider may help to smooth over some of the rough edges. If possible, include your mate. But once again, don't force the issue. It's better for you, at least, to get some counseling. If your marriage does end, outside support will be very helpful in getting you back on your feet emotionally.

What About Money?

Your ostomy can present added money problems, especially for your spouse. If you are the bread-winner, your spouse may fear the unpleasant role of becoming more responsible for financial aspects of family management. If your spouse is the major income-producer, pressure from the added costs of supplies and medical care may be tough. Both you and your spouse will worry about whether all obligations can be met (and continue to be met). Money concerns are frequently a major source of friction in any marriage. Here the problem is just compounded. Having an ostomy can be expensive, and this can certainly add to the friction. Sit down, talk it over, and be realistic. No one has declared bankruptcy because of an ostomy. Although new strains may arise, these things frequently have a way of working themselves out. Be patient, be communicative, and be positive.

Is Sex Affected?

One important area in which an ostomy may affect a marital relationship is in the area of sex. The chapter, *Sex and Ostomy*, provides more information on this important subject.

A Marital (Con) Summation

Coping with your spouse while you have an ostomy can be extremely difficult and, occasionally, impossible. Any marriage has its ups and downs, its problems, that have to be worked out. Having an ostomy makes relationships more prone to crises and arguments. Working through ostomy-related problems requires much more attention to your spouse's feelings and needs. But it's worth it. If problem spots can be smoothed out, your spouse can really be your best ally in helping you adjust to your ostomy.

COPING WITH PARENTS

Parents have a very hard time dealing with an ostomy, or any illness or condition, in their child (even in an adult "child"). This makes coping harder for you, too. Why? You don't want your parents to suffer or be upset. You'd probably feel guilty about their suffering.

If your relationship with your parents is good, then you're among the lucky ones. But what if you normally have difficulty dealing with your parents? Having an ostomy doesn't help. How have your parents treated you since your surgery? Do they ignore or minimize your ostomy? Or do they smother you?

The Ignorers

Fran, a 26-year-old dental hygienist living with her parents, had ostomy surgery less than a year ago. Since her surgery, her parents have been showing less and less concern. They don't ask questions. Even worse, they don't show any interest when she wants to tell them something about it.

Parents who ignore or play down your ostomy often do this because they can't deal with it. They can't accept the possibility that it might have something to do with them. How? They may be afraid that they did something contributing to the illness or condition that led to the surgery. Or maybe they think you inherited the surgery-causing illness or condition from them.

Even if this is far from the truth, it doesn't eliminate the worry underlying such thoughts. To avoid these unpleasant feelings, they may try to deny your having an ostomy. They might minimize it, hoping it will all go away.

The Smotherers

Since Louise's ostomy surgery, her mother has visited her an average of four times a week. This would be nice, except: 1. Her mother lives 30 minutes away by car. 2. Her mother has a heart condition and needs her rest. 3. Louise doesn't want to see her that often. You see, Louise is 39, hasn't lived at home for 18 years, and often disagrees with her mother's opinions (especially regarding what appliances to use and what activities she should participate in). Louise certainly feels smothered.

Parents who smother believe that, if you have any kind of problem, they must take care of you. Having an ostomy certainly fits this requirement. It doesn't matter how old you are, or what your marital status is. What matters to them is that they are your parents. They are responsible for you and must take care of you. The fact that you can take care of yourself doesn't matter. They'll call frequently, asking how you're doing. They'll want to know what they can do to help. They may come over as often as possible to make sure you're o.k. Whether they come or not, they'll constantly bombard you with questions about your health and activities. What can you do, short of moving out of town and taking on a new identity?

Remember what we said before? It really helps to see a situation through someone else's eyes! Don't you think this holds true here, too? Look at yourself, and your condition, through the eyes of your parents. How do you think they feel? What do they see? You don't have to agree with them, but understanding this will help you talk to them. Looking at your condition through their eyes will also help any discussions you may have with them, as you try to explain how you feel. It's fine to let them know that it bothers you when they do certain things. You'll feel great if your discussions are more productive.

What If Talking Doesn't Help?

If you have tried to talk to them and haven't succeeded, at least you've tried. That will help you feel a little better! At least you won't feel like you should do more—to convince them to switch to your way of thinking! What do you do then? Concentrate more on helping yourself feel better, regardless of whether they understand or not. If they're unhappy with you because you seem to be rejecting their well-meant intentions, so be it.

By the way, if you're unhappy with parents who are ignorers, you'd probably love them to smother you for awhile. And, if you don't like smothering parents, the thought of being left alone is probably very exciting. There's rarely a perfect solution. No one gets along with everyone all the time. Instead of complaining about your parents' faults, try to look at the positives in their behavior. You'll feel better about doing this, too.

How Much Should You Tell?

You know your parents. You know how they react to things. What would you really like to share with them? Would you like to tell them how you're feeling at a particular time? You probably know how they'll react to good news and bad news, and how they deal with unpleasantness. How will you handle their reactions? All these factors will help you to decide how much to tell them.

Sometimes, it's easier to talk with one parent rather than the other. You might tell one parent what's bothering you, and let that parent tell the other. For example, your mother may be able to get through to your father better than you can. This will help everybody.

You might wish you could share unpleasant feelings with a parent because of the reassurance it would bring. It's nice to know that you don't have to face something unpleasant alone. However, what if your parents can't readily accept your problems even if they wanted to? It may be more detrimental for you to tell them things that they can't handle. So don't impulsively tell them anything. Think and analyze. Try to understand what you want to share, and what their reactions may be. It's worth the effort. By spending a little time to figure out what's best, you can help yourself feel a lot better. You'll probably improve your relationship with your parents, as well.

COPING WITH CHILDREN

Children need a lot from their parents. This can surely be frustrating if you're unable to provide as much for them as you would like. You can't do as much, or help them as much. This does not mean that you don't love them or that you're not a good parent. Because each person lives differently with an ostomy, there's no way of predicting how long it will take until you can do more physically (or even emotionally) in raising your children. It may be hard to acknowledge your shortcomings as a parent. But think about your children. How much do they know about your ostomy? How hard is it for them to deal with your ostomy? Let's see how you can help them.

How Can I Explain?

The younger the child, the less of an explanation he or she will need. Anything that you tell a youngster will have to be explained simply.

With older children, explanations can be more detailed. Encourage their questions. Bobby, age 11, knew his father had an ostomy. But his father couldn't understand why Bobby rarely asked any questions about it. Was he keeping unhappy thoughts inside, or had he just accepted it and didn't feel it was necessary to ask anything? Remember: if your children really don't want to ask you anything, they won't. But let them know that they can if they want to. Upsetting thoughts kept inside can be even more destructive.

The questions of older children will probably be more direct and more specific. Resulting discussions, if handled properly, will not only be helpful for your children—you'll enjoy them! You'll also enjoy the great feeling of closeness that can result.

Fielding Children's Questions

How do you answer questions? This depends on the age of the child, as well as on how much of an answer the child may be looking for. The best advice is to provide direct answers to the specific questions. Don't go into detail, unless your child asks for more information.

Think, for example, about parents talking with their children about sex. Because of the delicate nature of the subject, and the discomfort or anxiety on the part of the parent, more information than necessary is usually given. Have you heard the anecdote about the very young child who walked up to his mother and asked, "Mommy, where did I come from???" The mother started trembling because this was the first time she heard such a question from her child. But she nervously explained the various parts of the female anatomy and how the sexual act resulted in conception. She told how this ultimately led to the birth of the child. When she finished after about fifteen minutes, she breathed a sigh of relief and expectantly waited for her child's reaction. The child responded, "But Mommy, I didn't want to know all that. I just wanted to know what hospital I was born in!"

The message in this anecdote is clear. Try to determine exactly what the child wants to know. Some children may not even know what answers they are looking for. So just start answering and then ask if that's what they wanted to know. Continue from there.

Be careful not to frighten your child. Children have great imaginations. You don't want your answers to get blown out of proportion. You do want your child to continue to talk to you about your ostomy. If you show that you accept the ostomy and the way it affects you, and you even welcome questions about it, this will greatly benefit the relationship with your child.

"Will You Die?"

This is an inevitable question. Whenever a child knows that a parent has had surgery, he or she may worry. You'll have to handle this very carefully. Children become petrified thinking about the death of a parent. They don't understand what you're going through and they will certainly be afraid. Reassure them that you're not going to die. These may seem like empty words, but that's what they need to hear.

It may not be enough for you to tell your child that you will not die, especially if you're not sure yourself. (Children are very perceptive: they'll recognize your fears.) It might be best, therefore, to speak to a professional (your physician or your child's pediatrician, for example) and include him or her in the discussion.

Should You Play "Show and Tell?"

One of the most common questions parents ask themselves is, "Should I show my child my ostomy?" For some individuals, this isn't a problem. They either know perfectly well that they will, or equally well that they won't. But if you're not sure and you're still questioning what you should do, then play it by ear. If your children keep asking, and you can prepare them adequately, then showing them the whole enchilada shouldn't pose any problem at all. It would probably be best to show them at a quiet time (not yours, the ostomy's!). You'll probably handle the situation even more easily than you anticipate. This doesn't mean, however, that you must show anyone. Use your judgment. If in doubt, check it out. Ask a professional, or someone else whose opinion you respect.

Spending Time

One of the hardest parts of coping with children is handling their disappointment when you can't do all that they'd like you to do. You want to be a good parent. But what does that entail? Most parents believe that they must spend lots of time with their children, taking them places, doing things with them. If this doesn't happen, parents may feel guilty. But ostomy surgery may temporarily prevent you from doing a lot of what you'd like to do. You have no choice. How do you solve this dilemma? How do you explain to your child that you can't take him or her somewhere, or that you can't do what you had promised? Children don't want to understand when they're upset. Making deals can help. Explain to your children that right now you're not strong enough to do much. Come to an agreement with them about some enjoyable activity you can do together when you're feeling better. This arrangement will show your children that you're aware of their unhappiness and want to help.

Try to spend "quality" time with your children—special time when you really share feelings and activities. You shouldn't be as concerned about "quantity" time—the number of minutes or hours you spend with them. If your time together is precious, then this is much more important than the amount of time. Your children will do just fine. Talking with your children and being open with them is another important component in helping them to handle your ostomy.

COPING WITH ADOLESCENTS

Coping with adolescents can be very different from coping with children. Because adolescents are older and can read more complex material, they can therefore read most of what has been written for adults. They can ask questions if anything they read is too complicated. However, the main difficulty in coping with adolescents is recognizing their unique needs.

The Declaration of Independence

This is the age at which teenagers begin to assert their independence. Look out, world! The future generation is coming! Adolescents want to start moving away from the family setting and its responsibilities. Under normal circumstances, this can create problems in many homes. Your having an ostomy can cause even more problems. Why? Since your surgery, your adolescent may have to help out more than usual with daily routines and chores. At the same time, the adolescent wants to do less, and be away more. What a bummer!

For example, 15-year-old Douglas feels guilty about not helping out more at home, but feels that giving in is a sign of weakness (heaven forbid!). This causes Douglas a lot of anguish, which of course he doesn't want to discuss with his parents. The need to escape seems even greater.

So, dear parent, imagine how helpful it can be for you to be aware of your adolescent's feelings. Take the initiative and offer a reasonable compromise. Just showing that you understand will help. Maybe things won't seem so hopeless to the adolescent, after all.

The Need for Friends

Adolescents are usually less interested in spending time with family members, and more interested in being with friends. That should make it easier, but it may still be difficult for an adolescent to deal with a parent's ostomy. Even if the adolescent's friends don't know about your ostomy, the adolescent may be much more sensitive to the situation. Does this sound strange? Most adolescents want to impress their friends. Somehow, having a parent with an ostomy doesn't quite "fit the bill." Of course, there are some adolescents who are more mature and open about it. The extent of their love for their parent and a sound family relationship minimize the problem. They may sometimes end relationships with those friends who cannot understand the situation. Unfortunately, however, this is not often the case.

Another problem for your adolescent is transportation (that means you!). Many adolescents count on their parents to drive them to friends' houses, parties, meetings, and so on. But after surgery, you may not be able to chauffeur your teenager around as much. As a result, you may feel guilty because you're not being a good parent. Your teenager, thinking less of you and more of himself or herself, can become upset or even angry. Your teenager may also feel guilty, either because of recognizing this selfishness, or because of feeling like too much of a burden. The best thing to do is talk—a lot!

Talking to your Adolescent

Understanding the needs of your adolescent can open the doors to much better communication. However, if you want your talking to be helpful, you must treat the adolescent like an adult. This will provide the best response. Think about the concerns of your adolescent regarding your ostomy. Douglas may be very frightened that his mother is never going to get better. Therefore, he may try not to even think about it. However, reassuring him that your condition is fine, and that you're having no trouble with your ostomy, may help. If your adolescent feels comfortable talking to you about your ostomy, encourage it. But remember to respect the rights of those adolescents who would rather not discuss it.

Finally . . .

Your adolescent may shoulder more responsibilities because of your ostomy. This is especially true if your adolescent tries to deny your surgery. Some adolescents will be able to deal effectively with their burdens, but some won't. They may simply be unable to handle the pressure. If your adolescent must take on any additional adult responsibilities or jobs because of your ostomy, consider that he or she may also be ready to enjoy some more adult privileges and pleasures. How can you require teenagers to fulfill adult responsibilities and then restrict them to teenage privileges? If you're apprehensive about their maturity, keep in mind that if they're old enough to do adult chores, they might enjoy some adult privileges as well (within reason, of course). Adolescents will usually be more willing to help out if they know that they will be treated and trusted in a more grown-up way.

29

Friends and Colleagues

Aside from family, the most important people you'll have to deal with are friends and colleagues. Do we have any suggestions for coping with these important people? We sure do!

COPING WITH YOUR FRIENDS

Some of you may not want your friends to know that you have an ostomy. But let's assume that they do know. What are the odds that they'll know what ostomies are all about? They may have read about them, but it's likely that they've only learned about them because you have one! At first, they may have known as little as you did. Because they weren't physically affected, they couldn't understand what you were experiencing. Some wanted to learn more; some wanted to forget what little they knew.

Some friends may be very supportive following the surgery—maybe *too* supportive. Other friends may not be supportive enough, something that can bother you even more. Your own mood really determines their reactions. If you don't want them around, if you don't want them close to you, or if you don't want them asking questions and you let them know this, they will probably respect your wishes. But perhaps they won't be there when you really do want them around. It's important for you to strike a balance. You may simply want to explain that your feelings change and to please bear with you. You hope they'll understand the fluctuation of your feelings.

Apprehension Keeps Them Away

Friends may not know what to say to you. What should they ask you? How should they talk to you? This can cause so much tension that they don't even want to be with you. They may feel so uneasy that they feel, "Why bother?"

Friends may be afraid to call because they don't know how you're feeling. They don't want to run the risk of stirring up unpleasant feelings for you (or for themselves, if they don't know how to respond). On the other hand, there may be times when friends keep asking you how you're feeling and you would really like to be left alone. Many friendships are lost or hurt because of misunderstandings. These misunderstandings usually involve uncertainty on the part of you or your friends in approaching each other.

Showing Concern

Can anything be done, or are you going to be a hermit for the rest of your life? Don't despair. There are things you can do to improve the situation. Try to set up ground rules with your friends. Tell them how you feel. If you are the kind of person who likes to be asked how you feel, let your friends know. If you'd rather not be asked, let your friends know that, too. If your feelings fluctuate (sometimes feeling talkative about your ostomy, but at other times reluctant to even think about it), let your friends know. Your changing feelings may be harder for friends to deal with, so let them know that they should talk to you the way they really want to. You'll let them know if and when you're having trouble.

Clear up the question marks. If you tell your friends how you feel and what your needs and desires are, fewer unknowns will exist. The uneasiness about what to do or say, which can hurt friendships, will be reduced. Your friends will become more aware of your needs, and will feel closer to you and less afraid.

Changing Plans

Don't you love having to change plans with a friend because of ostomy "concerns?" Probably not. So you can understand how your friends might feel if they have restrictions placed on activities. This doesn't have to be so. Good friends, who understand or at least try to understand what you're going through, will probably be able to accept these changes. Others may be less willing to put up with them.

Asking for Help

As you recuperate from surgery, do you feel a greater need to call on your friends for help? You may need help cleaning the house, getting places, taking care of children, purchasing groceries, among other things. Are you becoming more selfish? No, but it may seem that way to you. The reality is: there are certain things you must take care of. So if you need help, reach out for it. You know this will not last forever. As you recover from surgery, you'll feel better and will be able to do more. But in the meantime, if your friends complain or show resentment, try to talk it over with them. Don't wait until a friendship is destroyed to realize that built-up problems should have been discussed earlier, when the conflict could have been resolved. If you try and nothing helps, remember this: if your friends still don't understand, what kind of friends are they, anyway?!

Asking for Help Appropriately!

If you do need help, figure out who to ask and what they should do. If your friend Myrna loves children, it would probably be better to ask her for help with the kids. If you know that Maureen suffers from "super-marketitis," requiring daily therapeutic visits to the local food emporium, then sending her for groceries shouldn't bother her at all. If Joe has a driving phobia, don't ask him to chauffeur you around. Try to arrange for a proper fit when you ask for help.

Older, longer-lasting friendships also tend to be stronger and more resilient. Older friends will probably be more receptive if you ask for favors. Newer or more casual friendships should probably not be burdened as much. Without giving a friendship a chance to become firmly planted on your hook, you may lose your prized fish—a good, long-lasting friendship. Don't come on too strong. You might say, "But can't they see that I need help?" The answer is, "Not necessarily."

Don't feel like you must do everything yourself. There's nothing wrong with reaching out for help. But you'll feel better if you try to evaluate who to ask for what kind of help. (By the way, when you feel up to it, a nice way to show your appreciation is through an unsolicited gift or gesture).

Losing Friends

What if it just doesn't work out the way you want? People you thought were your friends don't call or visit. Some are "turned off" by your ostomy. Others seem reluctant to make any plans with you, saying "let's wait and see how you feel." It's sad, but in some cases it just can't be avoided. It's not your decision! You may wonder if it was because the friend couldn't handle your having an ostomy. Was your friend uncomfortable being with you because of potential "problems?" Was your friend unsure of what to say or do? Whatever the reason, you've probably learned a hard, unpleasant lesson. Although you may feel sad, you can't change someone else's feelings. Be reassured that most people who lose friends because of an ostomy do make new ones. You really don't want a friend who is uncomfortable with you. There may be times, unfortunately, when a friend or lover cannot handle the ostomy and you may feel like you've been rejected. This can be devastating! You may feel that you have not only been rejected, but you will not be able to develop any other meaningful relationships. This is not true. You are the same person following surgery as you were before, except for an alteration in your body functioning. Keep telling yourself that so you can restore any confidence that may have been shaken by this unfortunate rejection.

Usually, however, if rejection occurs or if a relationship breaks up, it couldn't have been too strong to begin with. Many weak relationships have broken up because of ostomies. A sturdy relationship, even if it has to go through some rough times, will probably end up even stronger than before. Remember, you want a friend who likes you the way you are, ostomy and all! And there are plenty of wonderful, understanding people out there. So don't despair!

COPING WITH COLLEAGUES

If you were working prior to ostomy surgery, you should have no problem getting back into your job after recuperating. There are very few jobs that an ostomate cannot do. Precautions are only necessary in a job involving heavy lifting or construction work, which may put a strain on your abdominal muscles. Other than that, you can probably handle most jobs.

Where to Work

Five basic points should be considered when you are resuming an old job or taking on a new one. First of all, ask yourself if you feel comfortable doing the job. Do you feel physically and emotionally capable? Is it something you want to do? Your surgery may have made you more aware of your mortality. As a result, you might decide to start doing something you really want to do! Second, if you had been working prior to surgery, will your employer take you back? Or will a new employer hire you, given your present physical condition? Should you even say anything about it? (More about this later.) A third very important point is whether your colleagues will accept you. This, of course, does not mean that they even have to become aware of your condition. Many ostomates never say anything about their ostomies at work and nobody ever knows. Fourth, will your ostomy create the need for different bathroom procedures? If so, will this cause any difficulties on the job? A fifth factor that may relate to your choice of employment is the amount of stress involved. Was stress part of the reason for your surgery? Can stress exacerbate your physical condition? You may decide to change jobs if you recognize that your previous job was too stressful.

So you know you're going to work. You're going to spend several hours each day in contact with the people you work with. You will certainly want to feel comfortable around them. Let's discuss some ways in which you might encounter difficulties in getting along with your colleagues.

Employer Acceptance or Harassment?

O.k., your surgery has healed. You're ready to re-enter the job market. Now you'll worry about whether you should go back to your old job, or whether anyone else would even consider hiring you. What factors come into play? Among them are your prior sickness or absentee record, your present state of health, the possibility of prolonged absences in the future, and your prognosis for the future. The employer will certainly want to consider whether or not you or your medical condition will create any problems on the job. Morale, sick benefits, and liability concerns usually top the list.

The most upsetting cases involve employers who are unwilling to hire you simply because they know that you've had ostomy surgery. They don't even know what it is! If the ostomy has resulted from cancer, there may be fears related to this as well. At this point, you're faced with two choices. You can either give up and look for something else, or you can try to educate the employer (not with your fists!). This can be done through discussion, reading materials, or contact with a physician or E.T. If necessary, your physician can probably reassure your prospective employer that you're fit for the job and should be able to handle it in more or less the same way as someone without an ostomy. In addition, now that the ostomy has hopefully improved your medical condition, there should be a decrease in absences!

All this groundwork is frequently worth the effort! If you do get the job, your relationship will already be a good one. Greater understanding will exist. In addition, it's nice to know that your employer has at least some insight into your ostomy.

Now let's look at a different problem. Let's say that you already have your job, but your employer has been expressing his displeasure about curtailed work time. What if an ultimatum is given, stating that if productivity does not improve, you will be discharged (polite, aren't I)? This is another potential problem. So what do you do? You do the best you can. If an employer doesn't understand enough about your ostomy to know that you have some special management requirements, and shows little or no willingness to cooperate, then you're probably better off not continuing employment there. You don't want to look for trouble.

For financial reasons, should you wait until your employment is terminated? This idea has its pros and cons. If you receive unemployment benefits for losing your job, this could ease financial burdens. But if subsequent employers are reluctant to hire you because of the grounds for dismissal, is it worth it? Only you can decide, and you'll probably have to base your decision on your own unique situation. It's a very important question, since your psychological state is so important in your coping with an ostomy. If your employment is aggravating you, then changes may have to be made.

Colleague Conflicts?

There should be little for you to worry about as far as colleagues are concerned. For the most part, if you are comfortable with yourself, others will be, too. It's not as if you're going to flaunt your ostomy, making it hard for some people to deal with. Because it can't be seen, people who see you every day will eventually forget about it. They'll take it in stride, and won't even think about it. This assumes, of course, that people in your office *know* that you have an ostomy. But what if you don't want to tell anyone? Many ostomates don't even bother telling colleagues. Obviously, there is no requirement that you do so.

Would it help to provide your colleagues with some basic information on ostomies? It might, although it may not necessarily improve their attitude toward you or your ostomy. In addition, reading about something doesn't always lead to understanding. However, at least you'll feel better knowing that you've tried to help them understand more about your body. If they don't, they don't. Remember: you can't change somebody else. If a colleague (or anybody else, for that matter) can't handle or understand what's going on, that's his or her problem. You can try to open his or her eyes about ostomies, but don't make it your problem. If you've got an employer with an open mind, that's terrific. Don't be as concerned about other people who don't understand what you're going through. Concentrate more on doing the best *you* can.

The Bathroom

Of course, it would be best for you to be near a bathroom so that, if the need arises, inconspicuous trips can be arranged. This is necessary for changing appliances and releasing gas. But this may not always be possible. It then becomes your decision as to whether you'll let this inconvenience propel you to look elsewhere for work.

Fear Strikes Back

Of course, you know that perhaps none of these problems will occur. If they did, you might have a discrimination case on your hands. But who wants to mess with that? What should you do? Although there's no one best answer, you may be better off not telling your employer about your ostomy. If you feel that sharing this information would have adverse effects, maybe you shouldn't share it. However, each situation is unique, so you must play it by ear.

Time to Punch Out

Whether you need to work, or enjoy working, you'll certainly want to minimize any potential occupational problems caused by your ostomy. Take one day at a time. Don't worry about problems that have not, and may never, occur. If your ostomy does cause a problem, be precise in identifying exactly what it is, so that you can employ the best strategies to resolve it.

30

Your Physician

How do you feel about your physician? (What a question!) Some people see physicians as gods. Others feel that they're rich, unconcerned, cold professionals who don't really want to help. Of course, there are other opinions. What's your feeling? This plays a role in determining how your treatment progresses. You may find that your feelings towards your physician (or physicians in general) have changed since your diagnosis. Some people with ostomies don't have as much confidence in their physicians, figuring that, if their problem had been treated differently, surgery might not have been necessary. It may seem that physicians don't know best, and that you yourself know how you feel better than anyone else. Because of all these feelings, as well as the rising costs of medical care, physicians frequently bear the brunt of much hostility. But physicians *do* want to help.

OFFICE VISITS

Since you needed major surgery for your ostomy, and it resulted from some illness or condition, follow-up visits after the surgery are always necessary. These appointments make sure that there is no recurrence of the illness and that treatment is proceeding properly. They also ensure that the stoma is in good shape and functioning efficiently. As the period of time following surgery increases, so does the period of time between follow-up visits. Initial post-operative visits may be weekly, then bi-weekly, then monthly, then every three months, and so on. Eventually, you will see your physician no more than you would normally for regular check-ups.

Depending on your condition, the reason for surgery, and your physician, there may be different types of examinations during the office visit. Different tests are used to check on your health. Blood or urine tests are normal and will probably be done at every office visit. It's always a good idea to bring an extra appliance (just in case your physician wants to check your stoma and you can't put the old appliance back on).

When you go to your physician's office for a check-up, don't assume that everyone in the office is familiar with your medical history, or even with your ostomy surgery. By the way, this also applies if you ever have to be hospitalized again, for any reason! Let people know that there are certain things that they cannot do. For example, don't let rectal temperatures be taken if you no longer have a rectum! Usually, nurses should not do irrigation procedures, give enemas, or do anything with the appliance. These should be done by the physician. If cancer was the reason for ostomy surgery, treatment for remaining cancer cells will continue, probably using either radiation therapy, or chemotherapy. These strong medical procedures should kill off any cancer cells left in the body.

So check-ups are important to keep your condition under control. Although some patients deny the possibility of any problems and try to avoid check-ups, the intelligent patient goes for regular check-ups to make sure that everything is okay.

BEING AFRAID OF YOUR PHYSICIAN

Are you hesitant about speaking to your physician? Perhaps you're afraid of being put in the hospital if your physician finds out how you've been feeling. You might be concerned that your physician will not like the way you're taking care of yourself. You might be apprehensive that more surgery may be necessary. Despite these concerns, you do want your physician to do the best for you. So try to be completely open and honest about the way you're feeling and what you're doing.

STICK UP FOR YOUR RIGHTS

Patients like to believe that their physicians know what they're talking about. This doesn't mean, however, that you must blindly accept everything that's said. For the most part, physicians respect the patient who asks questions. Many physicians even respect patients who question their judgment. Disagreement doesn't mean that your physician will back down. But if you are unsure of why something is being suggested, question it. If you don't like a particular treatment, or if it does not seem to be working for you, speak up. Don't hold back. You do have the right to question.

GETTING SECOND OPINIONS

Because you may not absolutely agree with everything your physician says, and because no physician knows all, you might want a second opinion. You should always get a second opinion before surgery (unless it's an emergency procedure). But many people are worried about hurting their physician's feelings. Don't let that stop you. Think logically. Most physicians will accept your desire to get a second opinion. It will either confirm what they feel, or will point out the need for further discussion. If your physician objects to your getting a second opinion, you should certainly question why. This *does not* suggest, however, that you should make it a habit of going for second opinions. Nor should you continually shop around for the "ideal" physician. No such person exists.

BEING ABLE TO REACH YOUR PHYSICIAN

Want to get easily frustrated? Try calling your physician for whatever reason (whether it's an emergency or not), and having to wait long hours for your call to be returned. This may be one of your criteria when searching for a physician. Make sure you feel confident in your physician's punctuality in returning your calls.

After you've had your ostomy for a while, you'll better learn when you should call and when it's not as necessary. Certain symptoms, such as pain, or blood in your stool or urine, require you to immediately contact your physician. Other symptoms, such as diarrhea or mild constipation, may not have to be reported immediately. Discuss this with your physician. Find out his or her feelings about your calling if you have problems. Ask about the kind of things that should be phoned in. Also ask when you should call.

YOU'RE NOT "LOCKED IN"

If you are not happy with your physician, you're not under any obligation to continue seeing him or her. Don't continue a relationship unless it's a good one. Don't continue going to a particular physician if you're afraid to ask questions or if you are afraid to call if there is a problem. Don't stick with your physician if you don't have confidence in what he or she tells you, whether it's about treatment or medication. Finally, don't continue seeing your physician if you feel that he or she does not care about you and does not have your best interests at heart.

Your honesty is part of a good professional relationship. If your questions or disagreements hurt the relationship, or if you are afraid of being honest, then this relationship may not be the one for you.

You may want to discuss all of this with your doctor before making any moves. This might straighten things out and improve the relationship. But if it doesn't, remember that you're looking out for your health. You want the support of a physician who can meet most of your needs.

31

Comments from Others

As Ralph Kramden of *The Honeymooners* would say, "Some people have a B-I-G MOUTH!" You may agree with this when you think of some of the comments you hear from people around you. They may know you have an ostomy, but that doesn't mean they know how to talk to you about it, or what to say. They may say things that they feel are right, witty, intelligent, or even sympathetic. But you may think otherwise! There are times when a certain comment might make you want to implant your knuckles into the speaker's teeth! Or a comment might make you wonder if you're talking to a graduate of the Ignoramus School of Tactlessness.

But why are you reading all this? As you know by now, you cannot change other people. You cannot improve their lack of sensitivity or the way they talk. What you can do is learn how to cope with some of the ridiculous comments that you may hear.

ARE OTHERS BEING CRUEL?

Most people really say things out of sincere concern. They may be trying to make you feel better, show their support, or show an interest in you by questioning how you're feeling. Does that mean you must always be receptive to their questions and respond to all of them seriously? It would be nice. The problem is that hearing the same questions over and over can begin to get on your nerves. Initially, you may try to gently respond to comments or questions, or politely change the subject. However, this does not always work. Some people avoid this by simply not telling anyone about the ostomy. This is one way of coping, but then you'll always worry about others finding out.

For the purpose of this chapter, let's assume that we're discussing those comments that you can't avoid, from people who haven't yet learned to tune into your feelings. If you haven't experienced this, that's great! But read on anyway. You never know when what you read might come in handy!

THREE WAYS OF RESPONDING

Many of the things that people say to you may be legitimate comments, but may bug you just the same. Others may not even deserve proper answers. Still others may be said without considering your feelings. But it doesn't matter why the comment is inappropriate. What really matters is how you handle these comments so that you feel comfortable. There are three ways that this can be done.

The first way is by ignoring the comments. This is not always easy, especially if the person is waiting for your response, or seems genuinely insulted by your lack of response. How do you get them to stop asking (besides buying a muzzle!)? Change the subject or walk away—ignore the question.

The second way is by trying to answer in a rational and intelligent way, explaining your answer, how you feel, or what the speaker should understand in a given situation. But now you may feel like you're banging your head against a wall. What if you just can't convince the other person of what you're trying to say? Such frustration can be painful!

What if the first two ways don't do the trick? There's got to be a better way, and there is. The third way is to respond humorously. What does this mean? If someone says something unreasonable to you, or asks you a foolish question that can't really be answered logically, you'll accomplish very little ignoring it or trying to reasonably explain your feelings. You don't know if your answer will be accepted or if the interrogation will continue. So, in many cases, the third option may be best. This is called "paradoxical intention." The idea behind it is that the person is asking or saying something that is really unanswerable. So you're going to have a little fun with your response. Let's see how it works.

HANDLING THE "BIG MOUTH" SYNDROME

What might you hear? And how should you handle it? Remember, the best response is one that will educate the "commenter." You'd like to explain your situation in a way that will allow him or her to learn something. But you're only human. So how can you respond when you get fed up? Read on . . .

"You Look Awful!"

It can be very upsetting when somebody says, "Wow, you look lousy!" You may feel lousy, but you certainly don't want to be reminded of it. You surely don't want to think that the way you feel is so obvious to others. You'd like to at least believe that you look okay to those around you. Even if it's said sympathetically, being told that you don't look well may be insulting. So what do you say? You might respond, "Thank you, so do you!" Or, "Yes, I know. I worked hard to look that way." If you're really in a cynical mood, you might say, "I know I look lousy. That comes from hearing people tell me this!" Of course, you could always say, "That makes sense, since I don't feel so hot, either!"

"What's that Bulge by your Waist?"

Few people are tactless enough to ask questions like this, unless they really have no idea about your ostomy. But even then, this isn't the brightest of questions. So how should you respond? How about, "My real name is Pinocchio, but it isn't my nose that grows." Or, "I was beaten by four pregnant gorillas and that's the last remaining bruise!"

Remember: for this approach to work best, you want to respond in a light-hearted way. This will show the person making the comment that you're fine, but you just don't appreciate what he or she is saying.

"Are You Sure You Needed Surgery?"

What if a friend finds out about your surgery and says, "You should have gotten a second opinion. You probably didn't need surgery." Besides retorting that you did get a second opinion, how else can you respond to this? You might answer by saying, "You should have heard what other parts of the body they wanted to work on!" Or else, "You're right—I should have gone to more doctors. The smell of the antiseptic waiting rooms excites me!" Or, "I decided that, when I found myself playing 'best three out of five,' I had gone to enough doctors."

"What's that Gurgling Noise?"

Again, you're faced with being honest or, if you're fed up, with taking the humorous way out. "That's my own internal version of the babbling brook." Or, "Do you know that there's an epidemic of hearing problems going around? The first symptom is hearing gurgling noises!" Or, "It's the latest tune on MTV. Haven't you heard it?"

"What Did You Do To Yourself?"

Some people are convinced that, whenever something goes wrong, it is a result of personal neglect. You meet a friend in the street who says, "If only you had eaten better, this wouldn't have happened." You could reply, "I had the surgery so I *can* eat better!" Or, "If you want to see what great shape I'm in, sit back while I clobber you!" If, after surgery, someone asks why you're walking funny, you might respond, "Normally, I walk better than this, but I just finished a marathon dance contest." Or you could say, "I injured myself kicking people who kept asking me what I did to myself!" This does not suggest that you be unfeeling in your answers. However, if you need to let the "commenter" know that you don't appreciate these questions, that'll do it!

"Can I See It?"

Some people are genuinely curious. But that doesn't mean you are obligated to reveal your abdominal addition. By the way, there are some ostomates who need very little provoking to pull a Lyndon Johnson (remember when he showed his surgery stitches on nationwide television?). But if showing others your stoma is not your bag, you might try saying, "You show me yours and I'll show you mine!" Or, "The gurgling noises you hear are my stoma's way of saying it would like some privacy."

"How Can You Stand That Thing?"

In response to this profoundly sympathetic expression of curiosity, you might want to ask what alternatives there are. Or you might want to point out your feelings regarding the alternatives, such as, "What goes in, must come out!" Or, "It's necessary to keep me from really exploding!" Or you might simply say, "I don't stand it. I usually take care of it sitting down!"

"You Had a *What???*"

Despite more and more exposure (poor choice of words?), the subject of ostomies still doesn't come up that much. Many people still don't understand what they are. If you get fed up explaining, you may want to get somewhat more graphic. Since this book has been rated "G," we'll leave the details of your explicit response to your imagination. But be sure to write in if you come up with some great answers!

How do you respond to somebody who asks what an ostomy is, having never heard of it before? You might say, "Let's forget we even brought it up. Then you can keep your streak going!" Or you could say, "I never heard of it either. How's the weather?" Don't forget: you really don't want to hurt your friend's feelings by saying something sarcastic. However, coping with others' comments can be one of the hardest things about having an ostomy. There are times when being gentle and tactful with others is less important than helping yourself to handle comments without becoming aggravated.

You won't always have to use this technique, but you may want to. You'll always come across someone who will say or ask something ridiculous. However, as you learn to feel better in your responses to comments, you'll find that you can handle them more calmly. You won't have to use sarcastic-type comments, and you'll have more fun with humorous, enjoyable ones. You'll keep people on your "friend" list, rather than on your "you know what" list.

OTHER LOVABLE COMMENTS

What are some of the other comments that you may hear? How many of these have come your way—"Is an ostomy contagious? . . . How do you go to the bathroom? . . . Why don't you quit your job? . . .Are you sure you can walk up those stairs? . . . Don't bend, you'll hurt yourself . . . Rest. Don't do anything . . . What did the doctor say? . . . What is the prognosis? . . . *Wow*, have you changed . . . You must miss the way it was . . .What's the matter with you? . . . Can I help you? . . . I certainly don't envy you . . . Your having an ostomy is the worst thing I ever heard!"

IS THAT ALL?

It would fill volumes to include all of the comments that you might hear from well-meaning friends or relatives. By reading these examples, you can at least get an idea of how to respond in a humorous way. Look over the list. Can you come up with some goodies? You don't want to be cynical or cruel. Rather, you want to show the speaker that you're feeling well enough to respond light-heartedly.

A FINAL COMMENT

One of the most common and most irritating comments that you may hear has been saved for last. Imagine somebody who is supposedly sympathetic, and trying to help you feel better, turning to you with eyes full of compassion and concern, saying, "I heard about someone who died after getting an ostomy!" As you turn to walk away, you respond, "I heard about someone who died after telling someone with an ostomy what you just told me!" You walk away, head held high and a smile on your face, leaving the astonished well-wisher behind you.

32

Sex and Ostomy

This chapter is *not* rated R, for Restricted. Rather, it is rated E, for Essential. Why? Having an ostomy can certainly have an impact on your sex life, if you are sexually active. This can have an important bearing on the closeness of your relationship. What kind of sexual relationship did you have before you were diagnosed? (I'm not being nosy. You don't have to write and tell me!) Was it a solid one, or was it on shaky ground? This can give you a clue as to what may happen after your surgery, and you don't want it to get worse! If you had a good sexual relationship, you'll have an easier time getting over obstacles that the ostomy has thrown into your sex life. If your sexual relationship wasn't good, it is unlikely that having an ostomy will make it better. You may need some professional help to keep things from breaking down altogether. But all hope is not lost. If you unite with your partner to work things out together, reassuring each other, relearning how to please each other, showing a desire for each other, progress can certainly be made.

Let's get into the major concerns. Will your sex life change because of the ostomy? If you fear that it will, your initial reaction may be to never let anybody get close to you again. These concerns are most prevalent in the minds of single ostomates, those who have not yet developed long-lasting relationships. They fear that they may never be able to develop anything meaningful. Married ostomates, on the other hand, have at least some hope that, in time, their spouses will be able to adjust to their ostomies and their intimate lives can continue almost as before.

For most ostomates, sex can be as good following recovery from surgery as it was before. If you had surgery as treatment for Crohn's disease or chronic ulcerative colitis, for example, sex can be even better! Think of sex without abdominal pain or without apprehension about dashes to the bathroom. What a relief!

WHEN CAN SEX BE RESUMED?

Most physicians believe that, as soon as any abdominal incisions heal, you can get back into the act. This may occur within a few short weeks. In the meantime, this does not mean that there can be no intimate contact. Holding, touching, and sharing warmth with your partner can certainly occur as soon as you have privacy. But what if you are reluctant for full sexual activity when the doctor gives you the green light? You or your partner may be holding back. The first sexual experience following this, therefore, may be somewhat unpleasant. If you can't perform, you may fear that there is a physiological problem that was caused by the surgery rather than a psychological problem related to your emotional reaction or concern.

WHERE'S THE PROBLEM?

Let's talk about what the problems might be. There can be both physiological and psychological reasons for changes in your sexual appetite. Physiological problems are better suited for specific treatments. Psychological problems are harder to deal with (ah, there's the rub). Let's explore some of the different possibilities.

The Body Beautiful? (Physical Problems)

Can physical problems alter your interest in sex? You bet your hormones they can!

Physiological difficulties lead to sexual problems. There are different reasons for sexual difficulties following ostomy surgery. For women, painful intercourse may result from surgery removing the rectum. This pain usually diminishes in time as the rectum heals. Fortunately, therefore, this should only be a temporary problem. But while it is a problem, what should you do? Use soothing lotions. Lubricate the vagina thoroughly. Try different positions to see what feels the most comfortable. Be sure to use gentleness, caring, concern, and patience during your intimate moments.

Other post-surgical discomfort can also interfere. But time helps. Keep some warmth and intimacy in your relationship, even if other activities are less desirable. Don't be reluctant to tell your partner what feels good and what doesn't.

For men, erectile dysfunctions may be the most common problem experienced, even though this only occurs in a small percentage of cases. Physiologically, the location of the surgery, including possible surgery-causing damage, may lead to erectile problems. In many cases this is temporary. But it may take some time before nerve damage heals so that erections can occur once again. More radical surgery, usually cancer-related, can cause erectile difficulties. In some cases, surgery may result in the permanent inability to achieve an erection. Although having a permanent erectile dysfunction may sound traumatic, there are some men who don't even mind it that much. You can certainly have a warm, loving relationship where other feelings of intimacy can still be enjoyed.

If, on the other hand, the ostomate is not willing to accept a permanent erectile dysfunction, another possibility is prosthetics. The most common one is the penile implant. There are two basic types of penile implants. One is the semi-rigid rod which, when inserted inside the penis, maintains a permanent state of partial erection. This may be good for sexual activity, but not as good for wearing clothes comfortably. The other type is the inflatable penile prosthesis. This is an inserted device that inflates or deflates by squeezing a pump surgically placed inside the testicles. These devices may not sound like the most desirable additions to your genitalia, guys, but being able to perform sexually may make them more attractive. Working in consultation with urologists will usually help determine what type of artificial device is most appropriate and what ways it can help.

The fact that occasional erectile dysfunction may occur does not mean that orgasm cannot occur. If orgasm occurs, pregnancy can occur, so use adequate protection (unless you're willing to risk an unwanted pregnancy).

Other physical problems can affect either men or women. Fatigue can be a factor. If you're tired, you're going to be less interested in sexual activity. This can be a real headache! (Sorry about that!) Decreased sexual activity may not be a very pleasant thing to contemplate, especially if either you or your spouse used to have a "normal" sex drive. But if you're uncomfortable or fatigued, hanky-panky will just have to be put on hold. Is this a poor choice of words? Actually, it may be an excellent idea. After all, just holding each other can be a wonderful experience, too!

What about medication? Some can have an effect on sexual desire. Certain medication, such as tranquilizers, which reduce your anxiety, can also suppress sexual desire or your ability to achieve orgasm. The use of alcohol is notorious in reducing sexual abilities because of its effect on the body.

Going Out of your Head? (Psychological Problems)

Your body isn't the only thing that may affect your sexual interest. Your mind also comes into the picture.

What's the most important sex organ? Think hard now. The correct response is: your brain! (Did I catch you?) If a sexual problem exists that is not physiological, then it doesn't exist in the body, but in the mind.

A common psychological reason for reduced sexual activity is an altered body image. The loss of satisfaction with your own body can decrease your self-esteem. You may feel reluctant to share your body with your spouse or partner. Do you see your body in a distorted way? You may fear that your partner is less interested in sex because of the way you look. Actually, your partner may not feel this way. But you may try to avoid it, rather than risk rejection.

Having an ostomy may affect your self-esteem. Do you like yourself less because of it? If you feel this way, you may be more fearful of rejection by your partner. Once again, you may reduce sexual activity simply to minimize the chances of rejection.

Maybe you're afraid of getting pregnant. If this is true, it may be hard for you to enjoy sex spontaneously. Having an ostomy can make this fear even greater. Why? You may be concerned that having an ostomy will interfere with a normal pregnancy or childbirth. This, however, should not be a concern.

Sexual activity may be restricted psychologically, because of depression. Perhaps you're so withdrawn that you've simply got no interest. Anxiety, whether it concerns sex itself, the intimacy of your relationship, odor, leakage, or performance, can also hold you back. You may be afraid that you just can't "make it." Fatigue or exhaustion can be a problem. If you attempt full sexual activities before regaining enough strength, this weakness may interfere with your sexual performance. Sexual prowess can also be related to a loss or decrease in communication effectiveness. Any of these things can happen after any surgery, not just ostomy surgery. But they can also be changed with proper awareness, interaction, improved communication, and therapy (if necessary).

WHAT TO DO?

The best way to cope with this is to begin very, very slowly. Start off by talking, laughing, and feeling close to the person you are with. Becoming more intimate gradually is a good way to minimize problems.

The return to sex can be extremely pleasurable or extremely disappointing, depending on the participant's point of view. If you were looking for skyrockets, but were very nervous, maybe you were disappointed. But that doesn't mean it is always going to be this way. Once some of your concerns have been alleviated, you can be more spontaneous. This can bring about lots of pleasure.

One of the most important factors necessary for enjoying sexual intimacy is probably the ability to like yourself. You'll want to work on this. Feeling good about yourself and your body are very important if you want to enjoy your sexual relationships. In addition, this will make your partner feel more comfortable. On the other hand, if you don't feel good about yourself, your partner will sense this as well and may lose feelings for you. This can certainly interfere with closeness.

Talk it Over

A very important part of sexual relationships is communication. If you and your partner can share thoughts and feelings, you'll be in much better shape to work out any sexual problems that may occur after ostomy surgery. If communication problems exist, however, difficulties may be very hard to resolve.

Try to maintain nice, wide-open lines of communication with your partner. Discuss any sexual problems openly. You may even want to discuss them with your physician or E.T. This will help you determine whether the problems are physiological or psychological. You'll then be better able to work on them.

Remember: having an ostomy doesn't mean that sexual activity must be reduced, curtailed, or eliminated! As a matter of fact, it can still be as pleasurable and as important as the partners want it to be.

All that has been said, of course, assumes that your interest in sex may be affected by your ostomy, and that your partner is suffering. But what if the opposite is true? What if you still have normal sexual desires, but your partner is the one who's afraid? Maybe there's a fear of hurting you, or damaging your stoma. Or maybe you're regarded as a fragile flower, easily broken, and your partner is reluctant to be sexually spontaneous. This must be carefully discussed. If one-on-one attempts at working things out don't help, don't hesitate to get some professional assistance. It's well worth it.

SEX, DATING, AND THE SINGLE OSTOMATE

Communication can be a very important factor for the single ostomate. You probably keep asking yourself, "When should I tell him or her? *Should* I tell him or her?" So what's the answer? Information about the ostomy should not be left until its discovery is imminent, but should occur earlier in the relationship. When the relationship seems to be really clicking, and intimacy is a definite possibility, that's probably the best time to bring it up. It's not necessary to discuss the ostomy at the beginning of the relationship.

If you are dating someone and are unsure of the best way to approach the subject, one suggestion is to be simple but truthful, and explain that you are an ostomate and you need to wear a pouch. If your partner is confused and does not understand what this means, you can mention that you needed surgery to resolve a life-threatening problem, but are fine now. The only difference is that there is a change in your plumbing: your colon and rectum (or whatever) was removed. So in order to eliminate waste, you wear a special appliance. Explain how happy you are that you are really able to do everything you want to do. You'll probably feel a lot better after this explanation. It should lead to even better communication, and you will be thrilled to answer questions openly and honestly. Maybe your partner will want to see the stoma. Maybe not. Does this matter? Not necessarily. This is an individual's choice. It shouldn't hurt a relationship. But let's be realistic. Does all this guarantee that your date is going to want to hang around? No, but it does give you a better chance. Otherwise, isn't it better for the relationship to end now? One other point. If a prospective date or partner cannot initially accept your ostomy, this doesn't mean that the relationship cannot succeed. Some people do need time to adjust to this news. You did too, didn't you?

SEX WITH AN APPLIANCE (KINKY, RIGHT?)

Most ostomates wear their appliances during sexual activity. Urostomates always do. Ileostomates do, unless they have a continent ileostomy, and colostomates do, unless they are using irrigation. For the most part, however, even continent ileostomates and irrigating colostomates wear some type of pad or covering over the stoma. This prevents against leakage and irritation. All other ostomates wear appliances. Why? Take a guess!

In addition to wearing your appliance as sexual intimacy approaches, you will also want to empty it. In this way, you'll minimize concerns about leakage or spillage. You don't want to have to worry about things that could interfere with sexual spontaneity. Wearing a fabric covering on your pouch can also help to keep you from thinking about your ostomy. Wearing attractive covers on your pouch may even be a turn-on!

Positioning during love-making usually depends on the desire of you or your partner, but must also take into consideration the location of your stoma. Stoma locations may create discomfort in certain positions. Experiment. You may even decide to go into research! (You see, experimenting can be exciting and fun!) What happens if the unspeakable happens? What happens if leakage occurs, an appliance shifts, or gas is expelled? Anything is possible. If it happens, the best way to deal with it is to try to have a sense of humor. An interrupted sexual activity doesn't have to be an ended activity. Spending a few minutes laughing about what has happened and cleaning up any mess can lead to even closer feelings and warmer intimacies. Does this happen only to ostomates? Of course not. Sex can be a gas for anyone!

If sexual difficulties do occur and you can't resolve them through improved communication or other suggestions, it may be advisable to get professional help. Sex therapy can be tremendously beneficial. Many of these difficulties can be treated successfully.

AND NOW THE CLIMAX

Because sex is such an intimate and important part of a marriage (or any serious relationship), the whole relationship can be affected when either or both partners feel there is trouble. Try to discuss it. If necessary, include your physician or E.T. in a discussion to clarify issues that may not be as readily accepted. You can still have a warm relationship even if your sex life is less active, but not if there are bitter feelings and misgivings at the same time. Understanding each other's feelings is a very important part of coping with an ostomy.

33

Pregnancy

To have a baby, or not to have a baby. That is the conception. Whether it is nobler (or safer) to have children may be a big question mark. Why? You may be concerned (and you're not alone if you are) that the ostomy will cause a difficult or unsafe pregnancy. It shouldn't. Will you be able to have children? In practically all cases—absolutely. Let's consider some of the questions that may be raised.

DOES PREGNANCY AFFECT YOUR OSTOMY?

Pregnancy can place additional stress on you, although it is impossible to predict what will happen during anyone's pregnancy. But it is unusual for a pregnancy to cause any difficulty for the stoma or internal workings (any more than it would for someone whose plumbing is intact). You may feel better than usual during your pregnancy. Or you may not.

Will your stoma change during pregnancy? Yes. This is normal and should be expected. Don't be concerned. As the size of your abdomen increases, the size of the stoma may change as well. It may become more elongated, wider, or change shape completely. You may then have to use a different face plate fitting or a different appliance. However, this is temporary and the shape will return to normal within a short time after delivery.

If you have a continent ileostomy, you should have no more difficulty with pregnancy than any other ostomate. You may need to drain the reservoir more frequently, though, since the growing fetus will leave less room for the reservoir to expand so it can hold waste. The intubation process may also change. You may have to change the direction in which you insert the catheter. This is not a problem, however. You should be able to adjust with no further difficulty.

DOES YOUR OSTOMY AFFECT YOUR PREGNANCY?

Stomas, appliances, or new waste passageways are not hazardous to your pregnancy at all. As a matter of fact, one fringe benefit of having a part of your intestine removed is that your pregnancy may be even easier. How? There will be more room for the fetus to grow in the abdomen! Also, hemorrhoids are a common problem during pregnancy. But if your rectum has been removed . . . !

Unfortunately, this doesn't mean that your pregnancy will be event-free. Other problems that can disrupt any normal pregnancy may still be experienced. Morning sickness, nausea, fatigue, and other discomforts, are still possible. Thrilling, right?

CONCEIVING

Will you have more difficulty conceiving because of your ostomy? It shouldn't make a difference. Some women have problems regardless of whether or not they have an ostomy. Physicians prefer that you wait until your abdomen has completely healed before you try to conceive. In many cases, physicians advise that conception not take place until a year or two following surgery, so that things are basically back to normal.

Another reason for waiting is that any nutritional deficiencies produced by the surgery itself or by the illness causing the surgery will also have a chance to stabilize. In this way, you'll be in the strongest possible condition for your pregnancy when it does happen.

When you and your spouse do decide to have children, check with your physician to make sure that there are no reasons for you to wait. Why might your physician discourage pregnancy? Perhaps your surgery was necessary on account of familial polyposis (remember, that's a hereditary, pre-cancer disease). In all likelihood, your child will have to undergo the same type of surgery before young adulthood to avoid cancer of the colon.

For this reason, you might decide not to proceed. On the other hand, you might still be willing to go through with this, if having children means that much to you. If you are a urostomate, you may also have to be more cautious. You want to make sure that you avoid any urinary infections during pregnancy.

IF YOU DO CONCEIVE

If you do become pregnant, it is important to remain in close contact with your doctor. This is crucial because you have an ostomy. If any problems do develop, you will be able to "nip them in the bud."

Although you may have had an obstetrician before surgery, be sure that he or she will take care of you after your ostomy surgery. Some may prefer not to treat ostomates and will suggest switching to a different obstetrician. Is this wrong? It may be undesirable, but you certainly want to know if a physician feels uncomfortable.

THE STORK ARRIVES

When the big day arrives and you're preparing to go to the hospital for delivery, be sure to take the appropriate information and supplies. Wear your Medic Alert bracelet. Information cards should be posted clearly so that the medical staff is aware of your ostomy. You don't want any confusion about management procedures (such as irrigation or temperature-taking).

ARE YOU PACIFIED?

As you can see, there may be question marks. The best thing to do is to speak to your physician. Discuss your case, as well as any potential problems you may face. Remember: in *most* cases, pregnancy should not be a problem at all. But take all factors into consideration. And then—good luck!

PART V

Living with Someone Who Has an Ostomy

34

Living with Someone Who Has an Ostomy — An Introduction

Illness or surgery can create changes in relationships. No kidding! If you live with someone who has an ostomy, you may have a number of concerns. You may now see that person differently. His or her ostomy may remind you of your own vulnerability. You may have been dependent on that person before—now you have to shoulder much of the burden. Although you share the concerns of the individual who has had the ostomy surgery, you also worry about yourself. If you have difficulty dealing with your loved one because of the ostomy, you're not alone. Often, an ostomy in a loved one creates a lot of ambivalent feelings in yourself. Concerns about the future, and about the person's health, may be troublesome to you. This is not unusual.

What if you feel anger towards the ostomate, not because of anything the person did, but because of the fact that the surgery has created changes? This is normal, but may still produce guilt. Why? Because this anger is directed towards somebody who, at the present time, is vulnerable and unable to defend himself or herself.

WHAT CAN YOU DO?

If you are close to someone who has an ostomy, you have an important job on your hands. This job is made up of many components, the most important of which is the need to be understanding and supportive. This is very important, whether you live in the same house as the ostomate or are simply a relative or friend. Remember: ostomates do not have it easy, but they'll have a much harder time if they feel alone and isolated.

LOYAL LEARNING

A great way for you to help is by learning as much as you possibly can about ostomies. You may have unnecessary worries if you don't know things about an ostomy that the ostomate does. For example, you may not understand when an appliance needs to be changed. The ostomate's explanation may sound strange. You may think that the ostomate is making it up. By understanding proper management procedures, you can better provide support and understanding.

LOYAL FOLLOWING, OR LETTING GO

Don't stay on top of the ostomate (Emotionally, I mean. Physically—well, that could hurt!) Give the ostomate enough space to regain control over his or her own life. Back off as the ostomate begins to take over more of the management procedures. How about doctor's visits? If the ostomate agrees, you may want to go along for the ride. There may be times when the doctor might want to discuss something with you. However, if the ostomate wants to go alone, and feels strongly about it, don't force the issue.

ENCOURAGE, DON'T PESTER

Encourage adherence to proper management routines. But don't badger. If the ostomate is not taking proper care of himself or herself, there is a limit as to how much you can do to change things. Should you tell the physician if the ostomate is not taking care of himself or herself? That's a hard question to answer. You don't want to overstep your bounds and be resented. At the same time, you don't want to sit back and let your loved one create unnecessary problems. This is especially true if the ostomate doesn't seem to care. Play each situation by ear. In deciding whether or not to say anything, you should discuss it first with the ostomate. Voice your concerns, mention that you're afraid of a problem becoming worse. Listen to the responses before deciding whether to carry it any further.

SYMPATHY?

Because of the noticeable changes in bathroom habits, you may sympathize with the ostomate. You may feel sad about what he or she has to go through. This may help you to provide beneficial support. But don't pity the ostomate. This can be destructive.

How about right after surgery? There will be times when the ostomate is so fatigued that little or nothing can be done. At such times, it is not appropriate for you to insist that the person get up and do something. That won't make him or her feel better! Try to help out. Try to reduce the ostomate's pressures at that time. See if you can take over any of his or her obligations or responsibilities; this will certainly make things easier.

At the same time, don't allow the ostomate to baby himself or herself. Try to make life as normal as possible for the ostomate.

DON'T BE EXTREME

Frequently, friends or relatives go from one extreme to the other. What does this mean? When your loved one gets tired, you'll help out. But when the person is no longer tired, will you allow him or her to do what is desired? When feeling better and able to do things, the last thing the ostomate wants is to be told to get into bed and rest. Have faith in your special someone. If the ostomate really doesn't feel well, he or she will rest. Otherwise, let'em be!

HOW TO RESPOND

Can you always be sure of the best response to the ostomate? You may feel that, at certain times, the best way to respond is with sympathy and understanding. At other times, the best thing may be to just ignore what's going on and walk away. There may be times when you want to joke about the ostomy. But there's no way for you to know for sure. You can't predict the needs of the ostomate. How to help? Lay ground rules. Hopefully, the ostomate will initiate this. If not, maybe you can start the discussion. Mention your concerns. Talk about your interest in being as helpful as you possibly can, and ask what you can do to help. Things will move more smoothly if you have a good idea of what to do and when to do it. Even if there are no clear-cut, definite answers, at least there will be some constructive communication. You'll be better able to handle future problems.

KEEP TALKING

It is very important to have open lines of communication between you and the ostomate. This is the only way you can really hear how he or she feels, both physically and emotionally. In this way, you can truly be of help. This doesn't mean that the conversations will always be pleasant. Talking about problems, depression, fears, or feces isn't very enjoyable, especially if you don't have any answers. But with good communication, any difficulties will be overshadowed by the feeling of closeness resulting from shared feelings and concerns.

The majority of this book has been directed toward the young adult or adult with an ostomy. These chapters, however, are designed more for the non-ostomate. This information helps you to see the ostomate's unique experiences through his or her own eyes. The next three chapters will help you to understand more about what children, adolescents, or "seniors" with an ostomy may go through.

35

The Child with an Ostomy

If a child is diagnosed as needing ostomy surgery, it is very likely that his or her doctor will immediately have two or three new patients: the child, and the child's mother and/or father. This may be only the tip of the iceberg. The diagnosis of a child with any serious problem can have a devastating effect on the child's family. Parents, siblings, friends, teachers, other relatives—all can be affected, since they are in contact with the child. The reactions of these significant others play an important part in the child's adjustment to this new situation.

THE CHILD'S PARENTS

The parents of the child will probably experience a whole range of emotional reactions. Feelings of guilt and intense anguish are not uncommon. They may feel that they have genetically transmitted the problem to their child. Perhaps they did not use the right physicians, or didn't take proper care of the child. "Is there something we could have done to prevent this?" parents may exclaim. All these thoughts are usually emotional, but can be destructive unless they are worked through. Parents should not attempt to communicate these feelings to the child. Nor should parents make the child feel ashamed. Extra attention to the excretory functioning can cause feelings of shame in the child.

HOW TO TREAT THE CHILD

You don't want to make things harder for the child with an ostomy. So don't behave any differently from the way you always did. Don't be more harsh and disciplining, or more lax and indulging. If you would really rather help the child adjust, then treat the child as a child, not as an unfortunate youngster with an ostomy. Parents: avoid changes in the way you raise your child.

Try not to show painful or unhappy reactions to the child. Imagine how the child will feel seeing unhappiness in loved ones. You can be sure the child will feel guilty. This will only make things worse.

Brothers and sisters at home will definitely be affected. The degree to which siblings are affected varies, however. This depends on how much extra attention the child with the ostomy receives, and how brothers and sisters react to this extra attention. Do the other siblings feel like they're losing time with you or other relatives? This can cause tension between the ostomate and your other children. Brothers and sisters may become resentful of the extra attention given to the affected sibling. They may not believe that the ostomy is such a big deal, but think that it is being blown out of proportion for extra attention. On the other hand, the ostomate may not even want all this attention. This can create guilt!

A CHILD WITH AN OSTOMY,
NOT AN OSTOMY CHILD!

Emphasize the child rather than the ostomy. It is better to think of or talk about your child as still a child—a child who happens to have an ostomy. In addition, try to maintain a calm, emotionally-stable home. This is crucial to keep the family together. It is harder to change the behavior of more distant family members. How can you keep telling friends and relatives not to bring gifts or shower extra attention on your "poor child?"

As we've said before, parents (as well as others who are close to the child) should learn as much as possible about the ostomy. The more knowledge you have, the more understanding you can be. You can then be more supportive of your child.

THE CHILD CAN HELP HIMSELF
OR HERSELF, TOO

Managing the ostomy should be done matter-of-factly. Make it a regular part of life. It's usually not a good idea to give rewards to your child just for following normal ostomy-care routines. You want the child to learn proper self-care habits, not to expect a reward.

Regular family habits should continue as before. You all have to learn to live with any restrictions that an ostomy may impose. Hopefully, everyone in the family, especially the ostomate, will feel more at ease with your child's primary physician. In that way, any questions or concerns can be dealt with. Your child, especially if very young, will be less able to understand the facts about an ostomy. The child may ask, "Why don't I go to the bathroom like other kids do? . . . Why do I always have to wear this thing?" Other questions may also occur. You want your child to be able to ask questions, even if you can't provide all of the answers.

CHILDREN DENY, TOO!

Children may try to deny some aspects of having an ostomy. They may not concentrate on proper maintenance routines, and not change appliances when they should. You want your child to do what's best. But there are times when children may be able to do more than you think they can. Often, you are more concerned about the ostomy than your child! Try not to be overprotective. However, you should still protect your child. Even when your child pushes too hard, try to allow the child to learn for himself or herself what can and cannot be done. In order to mature while having an ostomy, the child must be aware of any limitations that may exist.

"LASHING OUT"

Rebellion against authority is a normal part of a child's development. When it happens, be sure that you are ready and prepared to deal with it. At the same time, be assured that a child with an ostomy will probably not hurt himself or herself seriously with tantrum behavior. So deal with rebellion the same way you would if your child didn't have an ostomy. Ignore it, wait until the child has calmed down, and then talk to your child. Do try to minimize the physical effects of these outbursts. Try to keep the home environment emotionally calm, stable, supportive, and loving.

TAKING CARE OF THE OSTOMY

Children can start taking care of their own ostomies as soon as they are toilet trained. The first step is usually learning to empty the appliance. As the child grows and is able to handle more things, changing appliances can be the next step. After that, the child can learn to maintain the skin and check for any problems. The ultimate aim is for the child to be completely able to take care of the appliance by himself or herself.

36

The Adolescent with an Ostomy

Ah, the joys of adolescence! Adolescence can be one of the most difficult periods in one's life. Adolescents are swingers, not because they have such active social lives (although they may), but because their behavior and moods may swing so extremely, from the childish dependence of years gone by to the mature independence of adult years approaching. Adolescents are frequently insecure and unstable. The adolescent years tend to be sensitive ones. Resentment and rebellion may arise when needs or desires are thwarted. Closeness is also possible on those occasions when adult understanding is shown. The adolescent usually works hard to become more independent, and asserts his or her independence in front of parents. Adolescents want to be on their own. They want to be able to stand up for themselves. At the same time, they don't want to be too different. Ostomies can make them feel very different. This can create problems.

REBEL TIME

Finding out that an adolescent needs ostomy surgery can cause major problems. The natural tendency of any parent is to become over-protective when a child is sick. Adolescents almost always object to interference from parents. Why? Because the adolescent wants to become more independent. The fact that parents frequently have difficulty dealing with the need for surgery (especially ostomy surgery) in their adolescent will, in all likelihood, increase adolescent rebellion. Rebellion is a normal

269

part of adolescence, regardless of whether or not ostomies are involved. Parents should try not to be overprotective, but as tolerant and understanding as possible. In cases where the adolescent does something wrong, supportive discussions are more appropriate than put-downs and reproaches.

Rebellion may occasionally lead to more serious physical problems for the adolescent. Why? Because a rebellious teenager may be less diligent with proper ostomy maintenance. On occasion, the adolescent may deliberately try to make himself or herself worse, perhaps by not taking proper care of skin, not attaching appliances correctly, or not eating properly. The adolescent knows that these behaviors can be harmful. So what? Hopefully, he or she will learn (without dangerous consequences) that there are better ways to get through adolescence!

PROBLEMS WITH FRIENDS

Ostomies have resulted in reductions in friendships. This can be a problem for anyone, but especially for the adolescent. Making friends is probably one of the most important activities during the adolescent years. The adolescent may have a hard time deciding whether to tell friends, and if so, which ones? There may be concern that this information will hurt friendships, new or old. Parents need to be aware of this, so they can try to help. In rare cases, the adolescent might even want teachers to provide short lessons about ostomies, what they are and what they can do (after learning themselves, of course!). Hopefully, this will bring about more support and understanding.

EMBARRASSING!

Many adolescents are embarrassed about their ostomies. To an adolescent, any illness can be a stigma. Teenagers have to be "o.k.," or it may cost them friends (so they believe). What about the stigma of having an ostomy? Adolescents are at that stage in their lives when social relationships are the most important. They may be reluctant to get involved in physical activities or attend gym classes, where the ostomy may be revealed. They may not want to develop social relationships because of concerns about leakage, odor, or the possibility of intimacy. All this may create a lot of discomfort in their young minds.

It should, therefore, be up to the adolescent to decide who he or she wants to tell. Teachers should probably know about the illness, since the adolescent may have certain needs (changing appliances) or concerns (odor, gas, noise) that require more delicate attention. Why might the adolescent choose not to share this information with all friends? He or she might sense that, in some cases, friends would be afraid, upset, or even hostile. Some friends might ignore the adolescent, not wanting to be near someone with an ostomy. So let your adolescent make the decision.

WHO HANDLES IT BETTER?

Many adolescents with ostomies cope better than their parents do! Parents may feel guilty. They may feel that they could have done something to prevent it. Parents frequently feel that it is their responsibility to protect their child from harm, disease, or injury. Remember: adolescents can (and frequently *will*) have normal, active lives, despite having ostomies.

In cases where adolescents can't seem to shake their concerns, the visitor program is important. It is good for an adolescent to see another adolescent who has had an ostomy in "normal" clothes (how many adolescents do you know who aren't clothes-minded?), and hear about the relationships he or she has developed (need I ask about adolescents being relationship-minded???).

Occasionally, an adolescent may act differently with friends (and in school) than with parents or other family members. Could it be that the adolescent enjoys the protection and concern of parents? Maybe the adolescent puts on a different "face" with family than with friends. Isn't that frequently the case, even if ostomies are not involved? Adolescents may be more willing to confide in their parents than in friends. They don't want friends to think they complain all the time.

Some parents try to protect their adolescents by not telling them everything about their conditions. This is usually not the best approach.

Adolescents should know the truth, so they can take responsibility for their own management. Adjusting to ostomies may take a while. By restricting information, it may take even longer. Anger and bitterness between adolescents and their parents may seriously hurt the relationship.

QUESTIONING THE FUTURE

As the adolescent gets older, certain troublesome questions may come to mind. The adolescent may wonder, "Will I be able to marry? . . . Will I be able to have children . . . Will I be able to perform my job well enough to keep it? . . . Will I be able to make and keep friends . . . Will I be able to finish my education . . . Will I be able to function as a normal member of society?" These questions bother almost all adolescents. Having an ostomy just makes them more worrisome. The answers? As long as the new condition is taken into consideration, and lifestyle is adjusted where necessary, the adolescent ostomate should be in the same position to answer these questions as any other healthy teenager.

A FINAL COMMENT

There is one main feature that makes it easier for an adolescent to cope with an ostomy. Usually, adolescents who need ostomies have experienced prolonged bouts with Crohn's Disease, ulcerative colitis, or another condition involving a lot of discomfort. Therefore, surgery can provide great relief. Whenever the adolescent has difficulty coping with the nonphysical implications of having an ostomy, the realization that the improvement in physical condition can help to offset this may lead to easier adjustment.

37

The "Senior"
with an Ostomy

We used to think of a senior as a student in his or her last year of high school or college. It was a term used with great respect. Here, we'll use the word with even greater respect. In this chapter, a senior refers to either an older peson who has just had ostomy surgery, or a person who had surgery many years ago and is now older. Out of respect, therefore, this chapter will be directed to you, the senior ostomate. In addition, anyone living with you will also benefit from reading it.

If you are a senior, learning how to cope with an ostomy is just as necessary as for any other age group. There are differences, however, depending on whether you had your surgery a long time ago or recently. If you had surgery years ago, chances are you've already learned how to adjust to it. Does this mean that you won't have any other adjustment difficulties? Not necessarily. Although you may have adjusted well to having an ostomy, appliances and bodies change. Skin loses its elasticity, and becomes thinner and less fatty. It may also become more dry and scaly. All these things can change the way your appliance fits and your success in managing it. Because of these skin changes, you'll want to use skin barriers liberally, and take extra precautions in gently removing your appliance.

If you are a new ostomate, you'll have the same adjustment problems and learning needs as ostomates of other ages. Concerns about interpersonal relationships and body functioning may also arise. Because of your more mature, experienced view of life, however, you may not experience the intense emotional reactions that younger ostomates might.

How about body image? Here again, you may not go through the same kind of emotional reactions that younger ostomates might. But this doesn't mean you don't give a hoot about body image. On the other hand, ostomy surgery usually comes about with little advance warning. This doesn't give you much of a chance to adjust to changes in body image.

Adjustment may be the most difficult if your surgery was cancer-related. If so, it probably came on so suddenly that it was even more upsetting than usual. It is the element of surprise that makes this difficult, more than a concern with body image. This can interfere with otherwise good adjustment.

You may also be concerned about the problems created if you must become more dependent on other family members. After a period of rehabilitation, this may no longer be a problem. But at the time of surgery and immediately following it, you can't avoid this concern. This is especially true if you know of other individuals who have been placed in nursing homes or other facilities because they were unable to function independently. This can be frightening.

SENIOR MANAGEMENT

Are you having any problems managing the ostomy and the appliance? Management procedures may be more difficult, especially if other physical problems exist. What are the more common problems you may experience? It is estimated that well over three-quarters of all individuals 65 and over have some type of chronic problem that limits functioning. Does this include you? Conditions such as arthritis, changes in bowel habit, loss of muscle tone, and weight changes, may all make management more difficult. Vision problems can also interfere with efficient management. Problems with your sense of smell or touch may make it more difficult for you to tell if your appliance is leaking or if gas is escaping. You may not notice it, but your skin (or others around you) may. Check more often. In this way, you'll compensate for being less aware.

Don't give up. Explore as many different avenues of management ideas as possible. There is a lot of innovative equipment that can be useful in helping to manage your ostomy, regardless of the obstacles you're facing.

For example, magnifying glasses, lighting tools, appliance modifications, or other different types of equipment may make it much easier for you to manage your appliance, even if you are limited visually or manually. Check with surgical supply houses, especially those specializing in ostomy supplies or senior citizen needs. Or ask your enterostomal therapist. What a great source of information!

Do you have any memory problems? (You don't remember?) Occasionally, memory difficulties in seniors present a problem. You may not remember whether you changed your appliance recently. This is another reason why you should check more often! You might want to make a chart to record when you've changed it. Then you'll have only to look at the chart.

TIME TO GRADUATE

Even though you're a senior ostomate, you will still benefit following the same routines or guidelines as any ostomate. In other words, try to prevent any potential problems, exercise, rest, eat properly, stay as active as possible, and, most importantly, think positive!

Concluding Notes

Well, you've just about finished this book. Hopefully, you've learned a lot about how to cope with an ostomy. Although it would be impossible to include every possible problem ostomies might produce, I hope that what you have read will help you to develop your own strategies for coping. Because things change, and something that bothers you one day may not bother you the next (and vice versa), use the book as a resource. Whenever you have questions about how to cope with a certain aspect of your ostomy, consult these pages. If you have any comments, information you feel is important, or additional questions, feel free to write to me in care of the publisher. I'll be happy to hear from you.

Except for temporary ostomies, an ostomy is forever. It's nice to think that, perhaps in the near future, other treatments might be discovered so that this type of surgery will not be as necessary. Until then, look ahead, walk proudly, and enjoy life as best you can. I wish all of my readers the very best of health and happiness.

Appendix

For further reading:

Jeter, K. *These Special Children*. Bull Publishing Co., 1982.

Lazarus, A. *In the Mind's Eye*. Rawson Associates Publishers, 1977.

Mullen, B., and McGinn, K. *The Ostomy Book*. Bull Publishing Co., 1980.

For further information, contact:

United Ostomy Association, Inc.
2001 W. Beverly Blvd.
Los Angeles, CA 90057

(213) 413-5510

International Association
for Enterostomal Therapy
5000 Birch St., Suite 400
Newport Beach, CA 92660

(714) 476-0266

Index